BREAST MASSAGE AND ACUPRESSURE

FOR IMPROVED BREAST HEALTH AND INCREASED FULLNESS

By Alexa Reyna

COPYRIGHT © 2015 BY ALEXA REYNA

All rights reserved. No part of this book may be reproduced, stored in a retrieval system, or transmitted in any form or by any means, electronic, mechanical, photocopying, recording, scanning, or otherwise, without the prior written permission of the publisher.

DISCLAIMER

The content in this book is provided solely for informational purposes and is not to be viewed as a substitute for professional medical advice or to be relied upon for medication or treatment. Always seek the advice of your physician or other qualified health provider if you have questions regarding a medical condition. Never disregard medical advice or delay seeking it because of something you have read this book. Neither the author nor anyone else associated with this book can be held accountable or liable, nor do they take any responsibly for any and all damage, injury, or consequence resulting from any attempt to use, misuse, adopt, or adapt any of the information presented in this book.

TABLE OF CONTENTS

INTRODUCTION		1
CHAPTER 1 Breast Massage		3
CHAPTER 2 Breast Massage Techniques		7
Breast circles		8
Finger Swirls		10
The Claw		12
Knead Some Breasts		14
Diagonal Glide		16
Duration:		16
Upward Glide		18
Fat Brushing		20
Nipple Grab		22
Cleavage Glide		24
Cleavage Push		26
Breast Squeeze		28
Opposite Horizontal Glide		30
Breast Bounce		32
CHAPTER 3 Acupressure		34
CHAPTER 4 Acupressure Points		39
Tan Zhong Point - 膻中		40
Tian Chi Point - 膻中		42
Tian Xi Point - 天谿		44
Wu Yi Point - 屋翳		46
Ying Chuang Point - 膺窗		48
Ru Zhong Point - 乳中		50
Ru Gen Point - 乳根		52

CHAPTER 5   MORE ACUPRESSURE POINTS   55
Yin Tang Point - 印堂   56
Shao Ze Point - 少澤   58
Nei Guan Point - 內關   60
San Yin Jiao Point - 三陰交   62
Tai Xi Point - 大鐘   64
Jian Shi Point - 間使   66
Zu Lin Qi Point - 足臨泣   68

SAMPLE MASSAGE + ACUPRESSURE REGIMEN   70

INTRODUCTION

Traditional Chinese Medicine (TCM), developed over thousands of years of Chinese history, has utilized the healing power of touch for centuries. These practices continue to evolve today and are now practiced around the world. These touch practices address a broad spectrum of health conditions, including acute and chronic pain, stress, insomnia, breast problems, arthritis, headaches, digestive complaints, respiratory problems, etc. But in this book we are going to focus mainly on how these touch practices will enhance the overall wellbeing of the breast.

Breast Massage and Acupressure will guide you step by step in the ancient practice of massage and acupressure. These techniques are designed to increase circulation and energy to the breast area, resulting in improved health and increased fullness. Provided in this guide are 13 massage techniques and 15 acupressure points. Each technique and point includes detailed instructions and illustrations for easy understanding and accurate execution.

The information in this book is easily presented and organized for you to refer back to again and again on your journey to better breast health and fullness.

No matter your age or breast size, every woman can benefit from incorporating massage and acupressure into their daily routine.

HOW TO USE THIS BOOK

This book was created to assist you in developing a customized daily breast routine for increased breast health and fullness. You can create a routine with all the massage and acupressure points listed in this book or you can pick and choose just a few. They do not need to be performed in the order presented.

Chapter 6 contains a sample routine comprised of just five massage techniques and four acupressure points. This can give you a starting point or you can choose whichever massage techniques and acupressure points resonate with you. In any case, we recommend picking only a few to start out with. It is better to do a few slowly and accurately rather than rushing through and trying to complete them all. You can add more as you start making it a daily practice.

Chapter 4 details the top seven acupressure points for breasts. In Chapter 5, there are additional points that are also beneficial to the breasts. It is recommended that you do a few of the points from Chapter 4 at the very least.

Ideally, you will want to massage at least twice per day but if you cannot, don't beat yourself up for it, life goes on. Do try to make a conscious effort to massage every day, even if it is only once per day. This is especially important if you are incorporating these methods as part of a breast enlargement routine.

NATURAL BREAST ENHANCEMENT

You may have purchased this book because of your desire for bigger breasts. By using the techniques discussed in this book, you will notice increased fullness in your breasts with continued use, but to gain a cup or more in size, these techniques will need to be coupled with another breast enhancement method. These methods can include taking herbs like Pueraria Mirifica, or glandulars and even using devices like breast enlargement pumps. No matter what method you use, massaging your breasts is essential for successful breast growth, and acupressure can be done as an added bonus. For more information on natural breast enhancement, visit **www.growbreastsnaturally.com**

Alexa Reyna

CHAPTER 1

Breast Massage

Breast massage is a simple do-it-yourself technique that can have profound benefits for you and your breasts. Whether you are young or old, perky or saggy, breast massage can be beneficial to everyone and should be a part of every woman's daily routine.

Some of these breast benefits include:
- Relief of tension in the chest
- Promotion of blood and lymph circulation
- Aid in detoxification of body
- Stimulation of hormone secretion
- Enhanced chest elasticity
- Reduced sagging / increased fullness
- Aid in relief and prevention of breast duct blockages
- Aid in reduction and prevention of breast hyperplasia, lumps, and tumors

Another benefit of daily breast massage is it gives you an opportunity to get in tune with your breasts. Giving your breasts this attention every day will help you to know what looks and feels normal, and you will be able to detect when something is unusual.

BREAST MASSAGE PREP

Breast massage is virtually free and only takes a few minutes a day. You do not need any fancy tools to perform a beneficial breast massage, just your hands.

Breast Massage and Acupressure

When massaging your breasts, be sure to use some type of lubricant to help hands glide easily over the breasts. You can perform breast massage while in the shower or use products already found in your home, like olive oil or body lotion. Lotions tend to absorb quickly, though, so if you plan to massage for more than a few minutes, an oil would be a better option.

Some items you can use for breast massage are:
- Cocoa butter
- Shea butter
- Coconut oil
- Evening primrose oil
- Sweet almond oil
- Borage oil

You can add essential oils or herbal extracts to enhance your lotion or oil. For those who are interested in adding more fullness to their breasts, there are commercial breast enlargement creams available that contain herbal extracts or Volufiline™. Volufiline™ is a cosmetic ingredient that is derived from the Chinese herb Zhu Mu. It increases the size and number of fat cells to the area that it is applied. Volufiline™ is commonly used to increase volume in the breasts, buttocks, and lips.

PRE-MASSAGE WARM-UP

To get the most out of your breast massage, it is recommended that you add heat before starting your massage to warm up the breasts. Simply place a heating pad on your breasts for a few minutes. If you do not have a heating pad, place a damp towel in the microwave for a few seconds or use a re-sealable bag with hot water in it. The temperature should be about 100-110°F or slightly above body temperature. Take care not to make it too hot and risk burning yourself. Leave the heated item on your breasts for 3-5 minutes, remove the item, and begin your massage. The heat will help dilate the blood vessels and improve circulation. If you are using a breast enhancement product in conjunction with your massage, the heat will also help to open your pores so that the product is more easily absorbed.

INWARD VS. OUTWARD

Many breast massage techniques involve circular motions around the breasts (i.e. Breast Circles on page 12). The direction of the circular motion plays an important part in how that particular massage will benefit the breasts. Performing the massage in an inward motion helps to bring nutrients and oxygen to the breasts which is said to help increase breast size and fullness. An outward motion helps to move toxins away from the breasts and clear the lymphs. Outward circular motion is said to be a natural breast reducer.

Most of the massage techniques found in this book suggest inward motions. But before beginning your breast massage regimen, it is recommended that you do at least ten outward rotations on each breast to clear the lymphs and remove any blockages, preparing the breasts for receiving the full benefits of the massage.

CONSISTENCY IS KEY

Ideally, you will want to massage twice per day, once in the morning and once in the evening. If time is an issue, however, massaging at least once per day, each and every day, can still be very beneficial. The best times to massage are during or after your shower and before bed. Massage can help release tension and relax the body and prepare you for a good night's rest.

MASSAGE TIPS
- When performing a massage technique, be gentle on your breasts. Do not apply too much pressure; this is not a deep tissue massage. If you are sore the next day or have bruises, you probably massaged too hard. Wait a day or two, and then restart your massage routine.
- Avoid the nipples when massaging unless the massage is specifically for the nipples.

Breast Massage and Acupressure

- Do not rush through the techniques and sacrifice quality. It is better to do a few techniques accurately rather than rushing through them.
- In the beginning, your arms may get tired. Take a break for a minute or two then resume where you left off. Your arms will eventually get used to it and won't get tired as easily. In the meantime, tired arms generally do not perform the massage techniques accurately, so give them a break.

In the next chapter, we will discuss a number of breast massage techniques. They are simple to do and require less than a minute each.

CHAPTER 2

Breast Massage Techniques

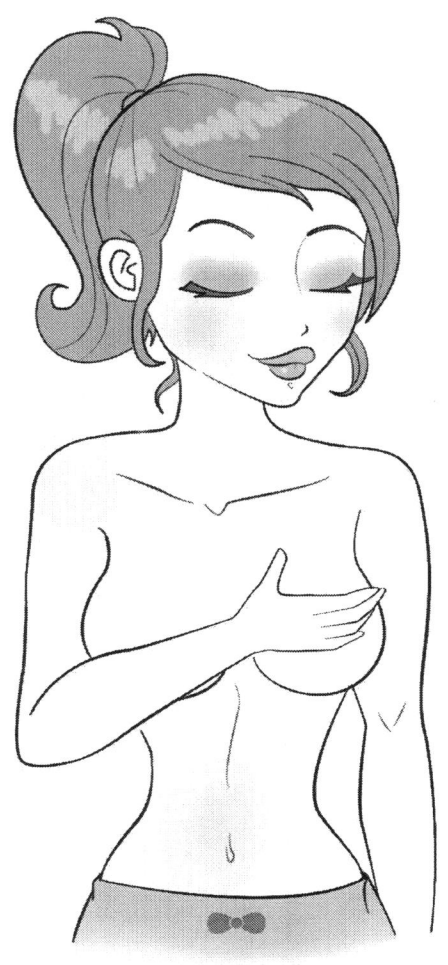

BREAST CIRCLES

Hand position:

One breast at a time - left hand on right breast, right hand on left breast.

Instruction:

1. Place four fingers on the upper outer corner of the breast near the armpit.
2. Use the fingers to draw a circle around the breast by going across the top of the breast, down the inner side of the breast, across the bottom of breast and up along the outer side of the breast (avoiding areola).
3. Repeat motion.

Duration:

Twenty rotations around each breast.

Notes:

Massage can be done simultaneously on each breast - right hand on right breast, left hand on left breast.

Breast Massage and Acupressure

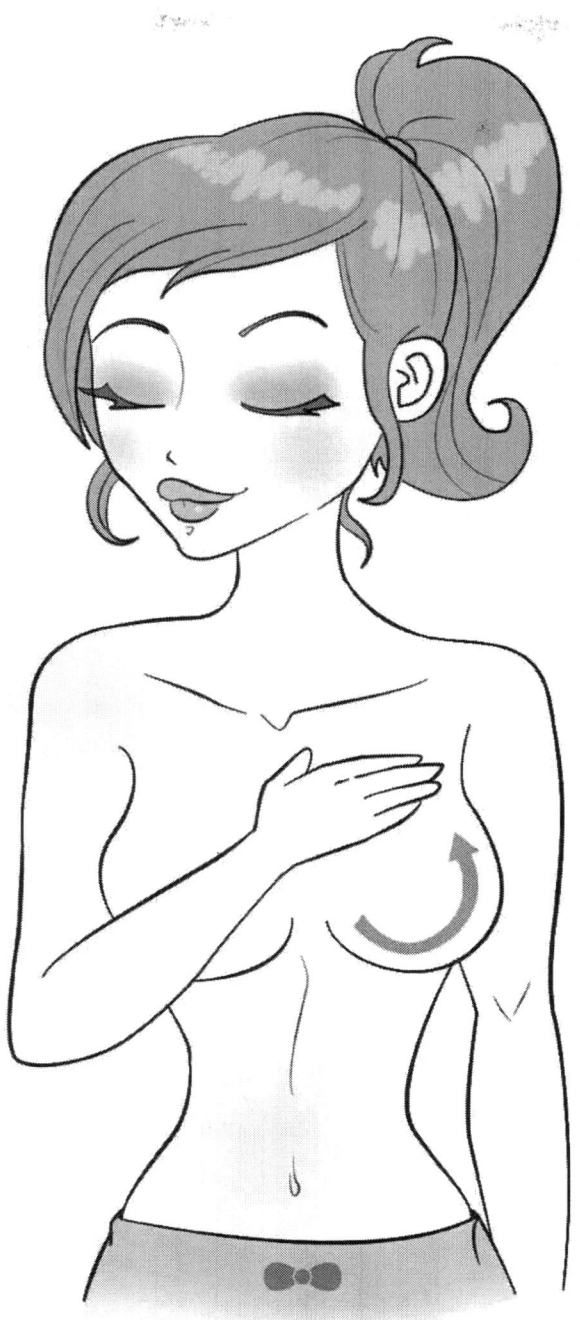

FINGER SWIRLS

Hand position:

One breast at a time - left hand on right breast, right hand on left breast.

Instruction:

(similar to Breast Circles massage)

1. Use finger tips to make little swirls in a continuous motion around the breast (avoiding areola).
2. Repeat motion.

Duration:

Ten full rotations around each breast.

Notes:

Knuckles may also be used to perform this massage instead of finger tips.

Breast Massage and Acupressure

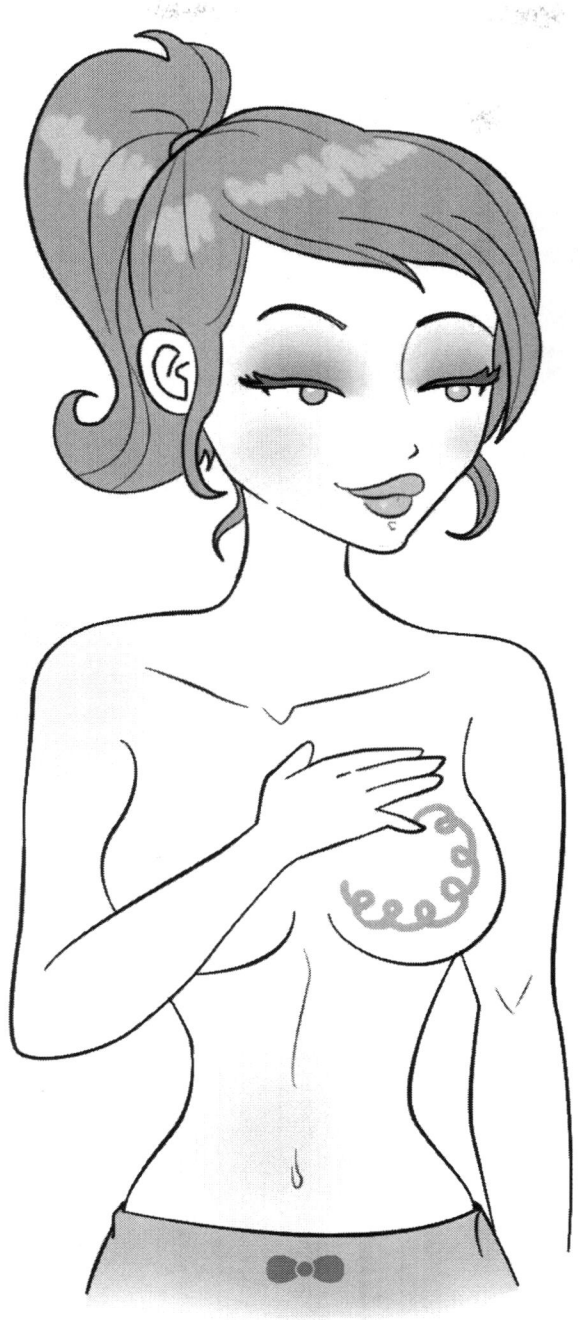

THE CLAW

Hand position:

One breast at a time - left hand on right breast, right hand on left breast.

Instruction:

1. Stretch hand across chest towards back.
2. With fingers spread slightly in a claw-like position, grab back and slide fingers across outer side of breast to the nipple. Stop when you reach the areola.
3. Lift hand up and repeat motion.

Duration:

One minute on each breast.

Breast Massage and Acupressure

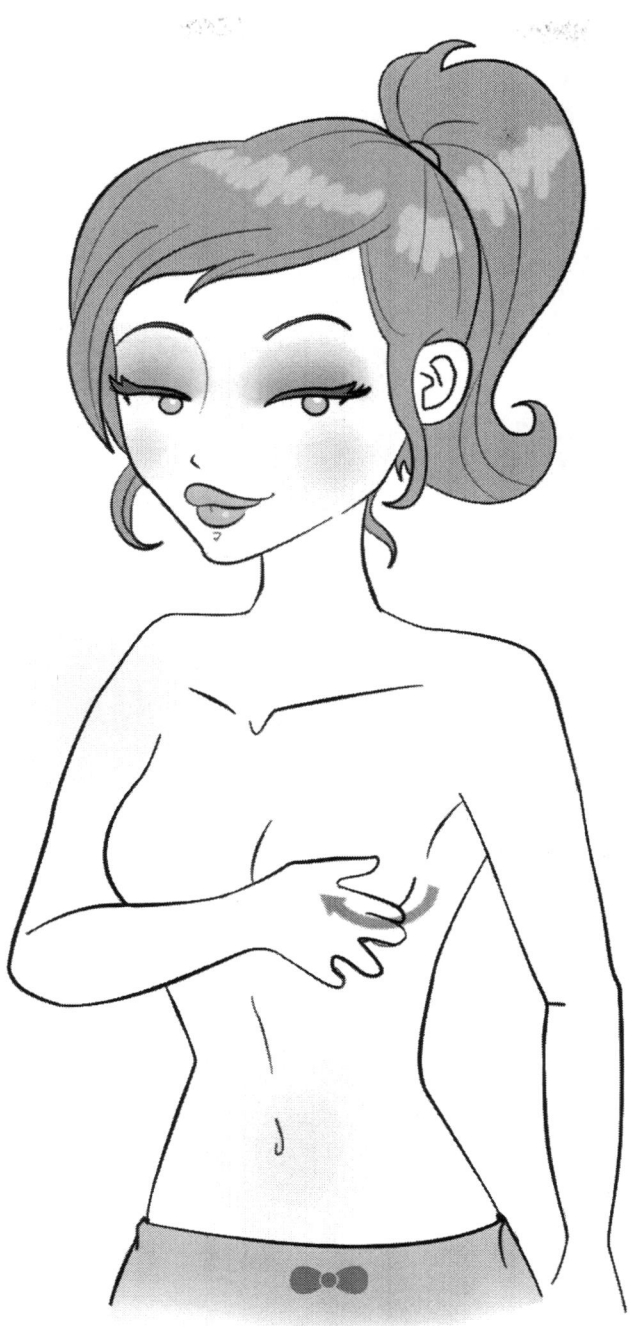

Breast Massage and Acupressure

KNEAD SOME BREASTS

Hand position:

Both hands focusing on one breast at a time

Instruction:

1. With left hand, glide from outer side of left breast towards the nipple in a horizontal motion.
2. With right hand, glide from bottom of left breast towards the nipples.
3. Repeat, alternating hands in a smooth continuous motion.

Duration:

One minute on each breast.

Breast Massage and Acupressure

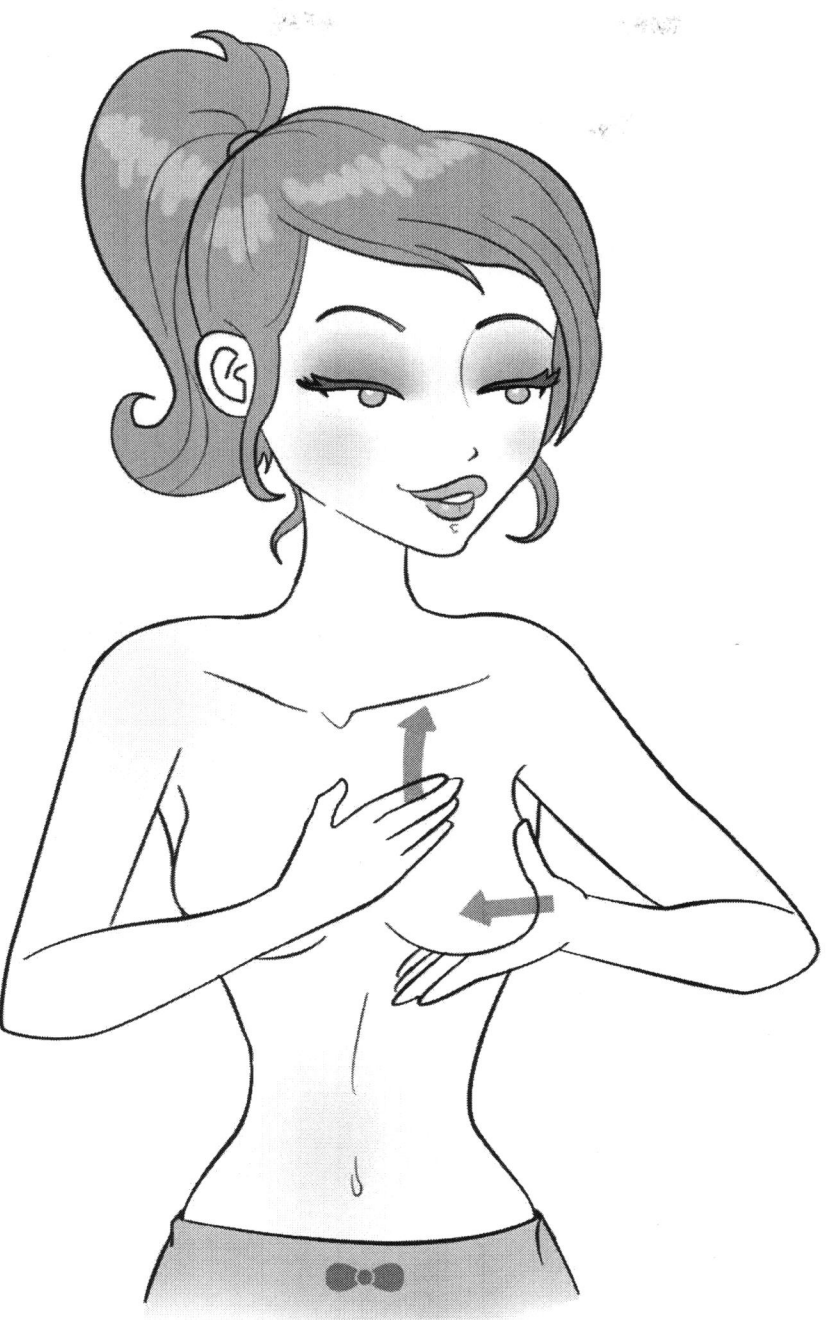

15

DIAGONAL GLIDE

Hand position:

Both hands focusing on one breast at a time

Instruction:

1. Glide hand from bottom outer corner of breast upward towards the top of the sternum. Stop at areola.
2. Repeat, alternating hands in a smooth, continuous diagonal motion.

Duration:

One minute on each breast.

Breast Massage and Acupressure

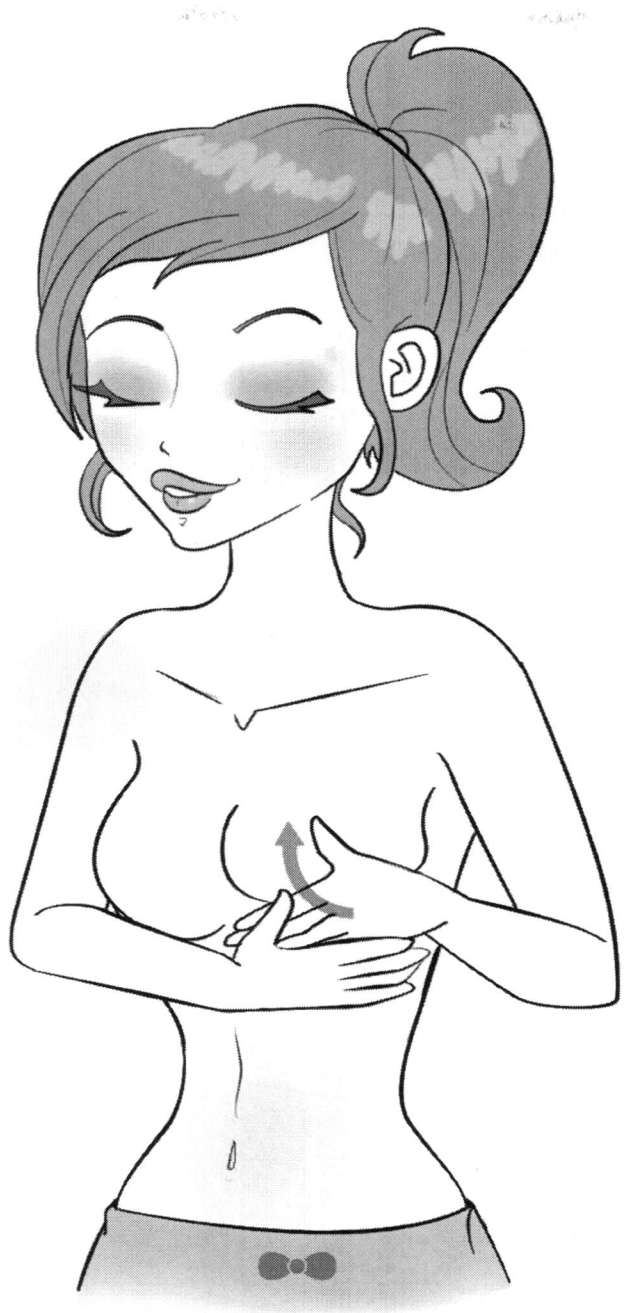

UPWARD GLIDE

Hand position:

Both hands focusing on one breast at a time

Instruction:

(Similar to Diagonal Glide)

1. Glide hand from bottom of breast upward towards the areola, stop at the areola.

2. Repeat, alternating hands on same breast in a smooth continuous upward motion.

Duration:

One minute on each breast.

Breast Massage and Acupressure

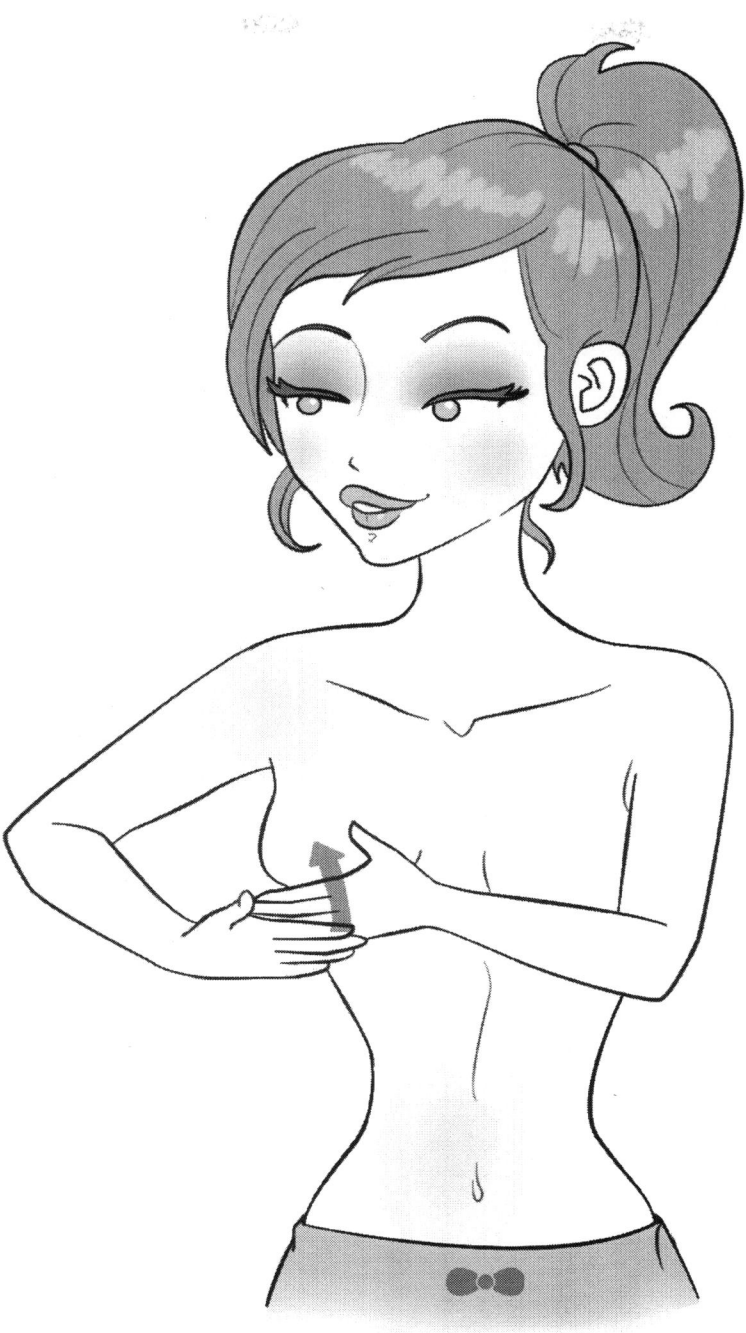

FAT BRUSHING

Hand position:

Both hands will be focusing on one breast at a time.

Instruction:

(Similar to Upward Glide)

1. Glide hand upward from lower abdomen towards the areola, stop at the areola.

2. Repeat alternating hands on same breast in a smooth continuous motion throughout the trunk of body, moving fat from stomach to breasts.

Duration:

One minute on each breast.

Breast Massage and Acupressure

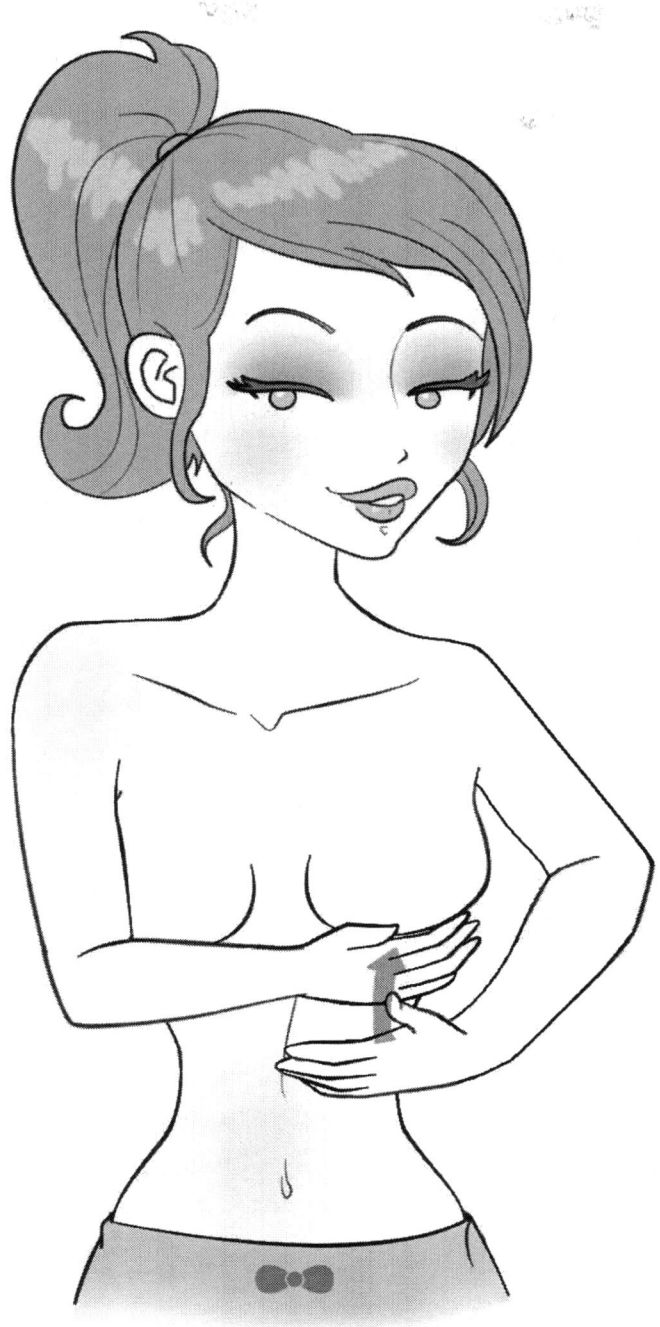

NIPPLE GRAB

Hand position:

One breast at a time - left hand on right breast, right hand on left breast.

Instruction:

1. Place all five fingers around the breasts.
2. Gently grab and pull the breast, slide your fingers towards the nipples.
3. Release fingers before reaching the areolas.
4. Repeat the motion.

Duration:

Ten times on each breast.

Notes:

This massage can be performed simultaneously on each breast – right hand on the right breast, left hand on the left breast.

Breast Massage and Acupressure

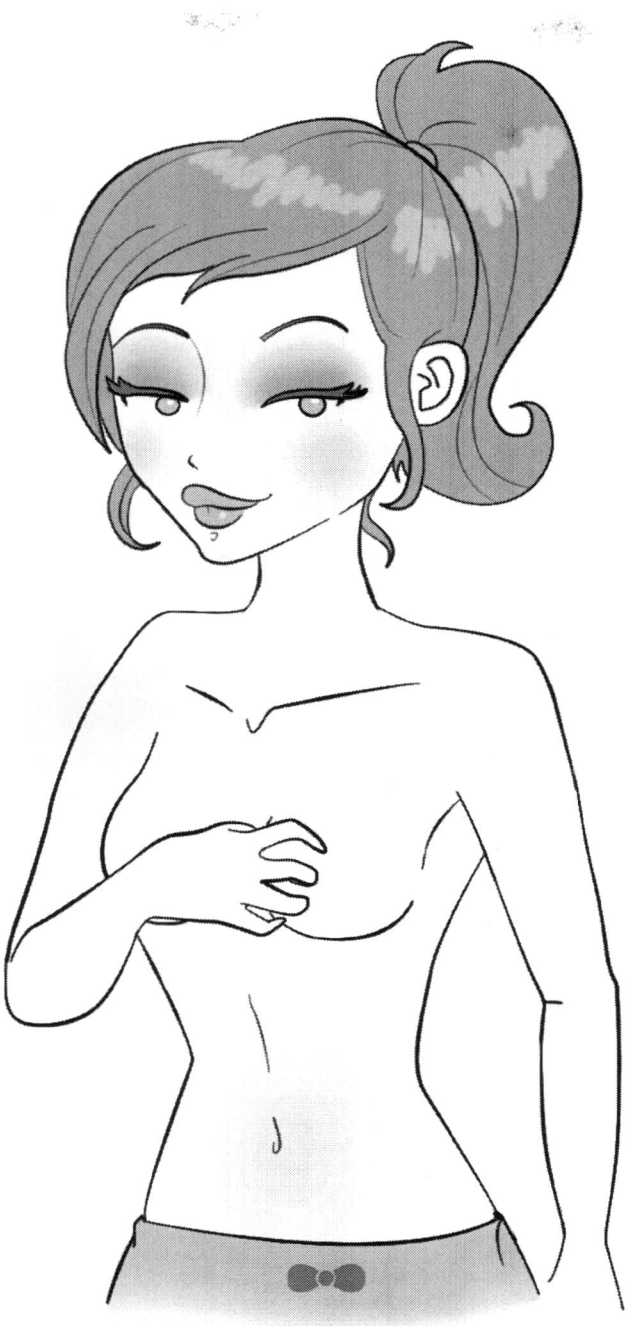

CLEAVAGE GLIDE

Hand position:

Both hands will be focusing on one breast at a time.

Instruction:

1. With left hand, cup the left breast and push up to create cleavage.
2. With right hand, gently rub the cleavage area from armpit towards breast bone.

Duration:

Twenty times each breast.

Notes:

You can use either your fingers or knuckles. If using knuckles, apply light pressure. Also, this is not a back and forth motion. When you reach the breast bone, lift your hand up and start from the armpit again.

Breast Massage and Acupressure

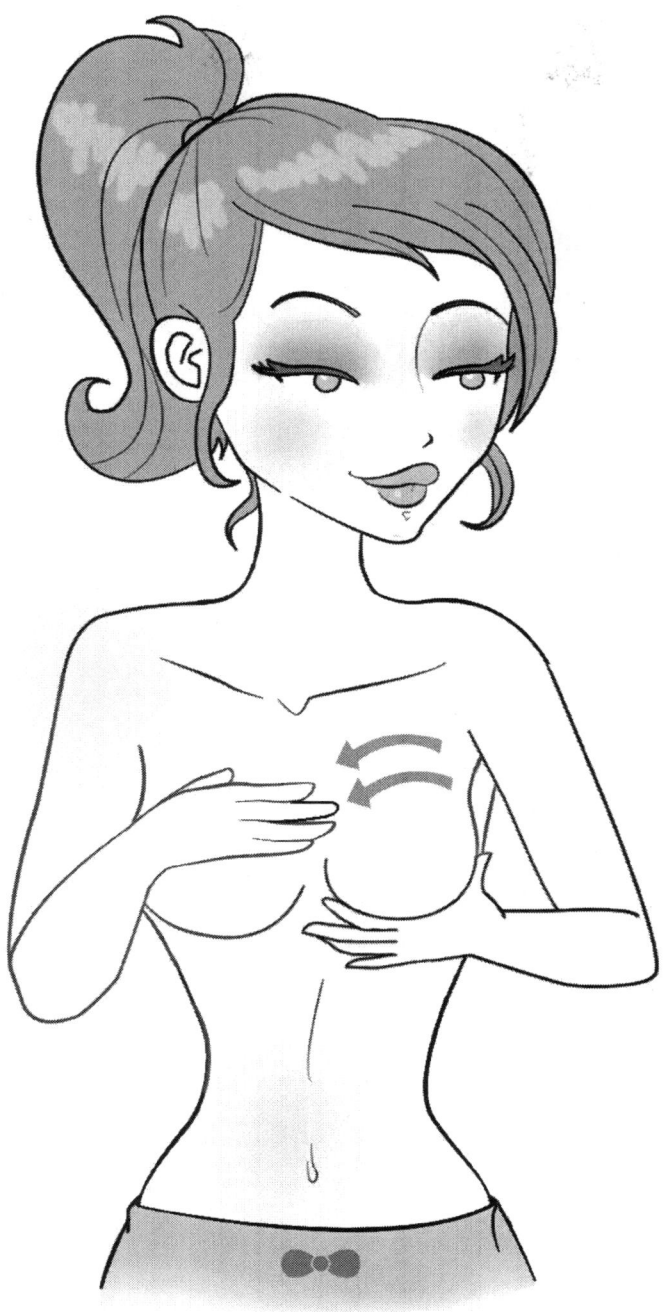

CLEAVAGE PUSH

Hand position:

At the same time - left hand on the left breast and right hand on the right breast.

Instruction:

1. Cup breasts in each hand.
2. Gently push up towards your chin.
3. Hold for a few second, then gently release.
4. Repeat motion.

Duration:

One minute.

Notes:

It is recommended that you perform this technique every time you remove your bra.

Breast Massage and Acupressure

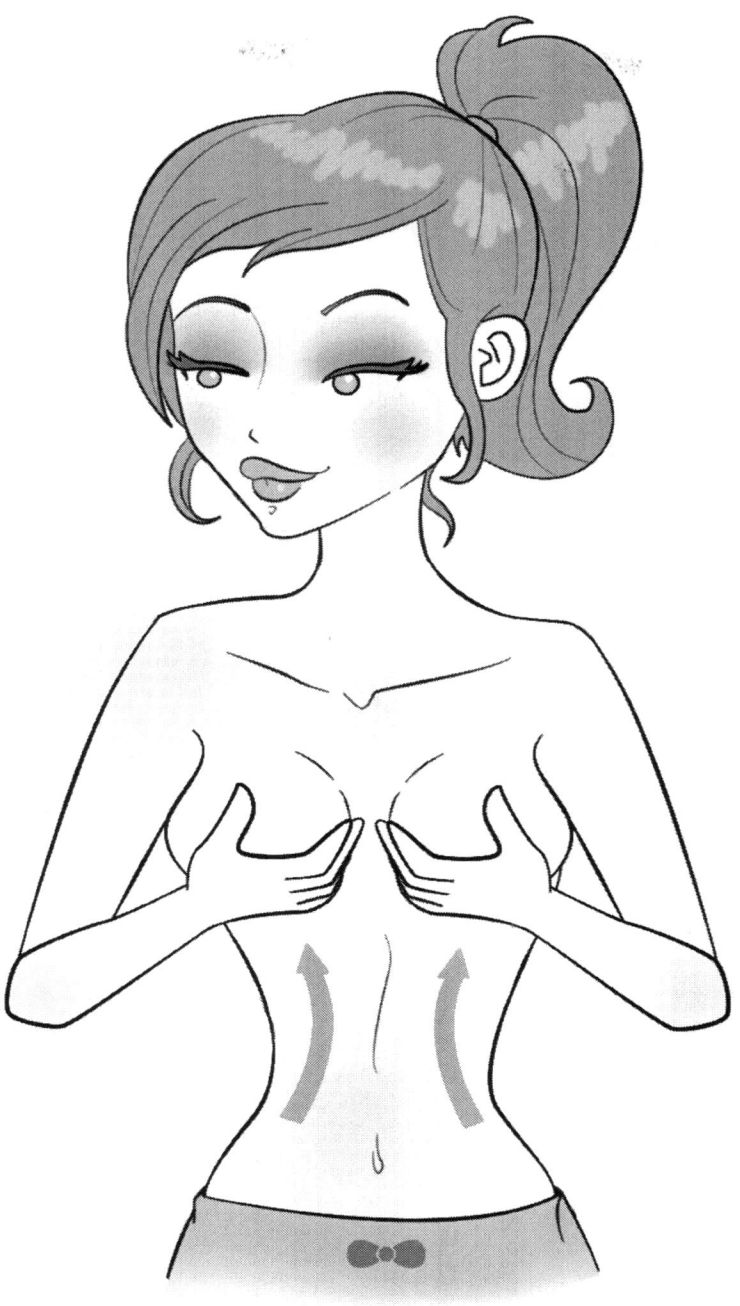

Breast Massage and Acupressure

BREAST SQUEEZE

Hand position:

Both hands focusing on one breast at a time.

Instruction:

1. Place right hand on top of left breast.
2. Place left hand on the bottom of the left breast. Hands should be slightly cupping the breast.
3. Gently squeeze the breast by moving right hand down and moving left hand up.
4. Repeat on the other breast with left hand on top and right hand on bottom.

Duration:

Twenty times on each breast.

Breast Massage and Acupressure

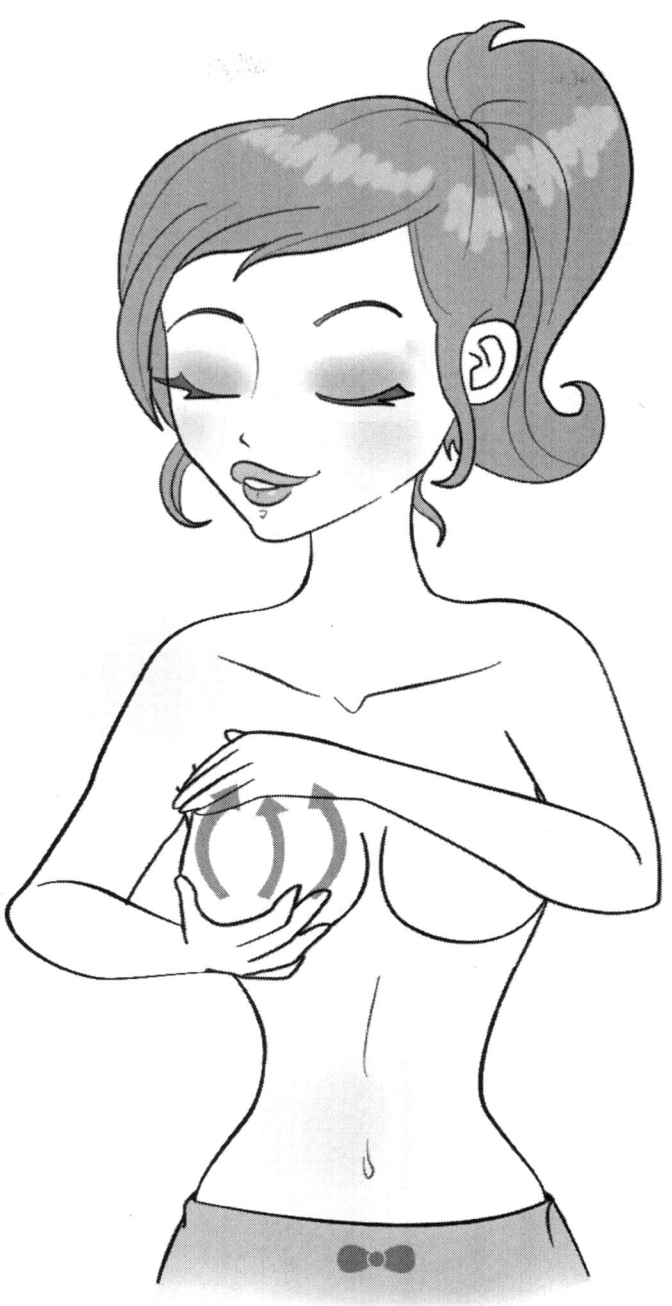

OPPOSITE HORIZONTAL GLIDE

Hand position:

Both hands focusing on one breast at a time.

Instruction:

1. Place right hand on top of the left breast and left hand on bottom of the left breast. Hands should be slightly cupping the breast.
2. Gently move the right hand across the top of the breast towards the right.
3. At the same time, move left hand across the bottom of the breast towards the left.
4. **Repeat motion.** For opposite breast, left hand on top moving towards the left and right hand on bottom moving towards the right.

Duration:

Twenty times each breast.

Notes:

This is not a back and forth (sawing) motion. After motion is complete, lift hands and place in original starting position then repeat motion.

Breast Massage and Acupressure

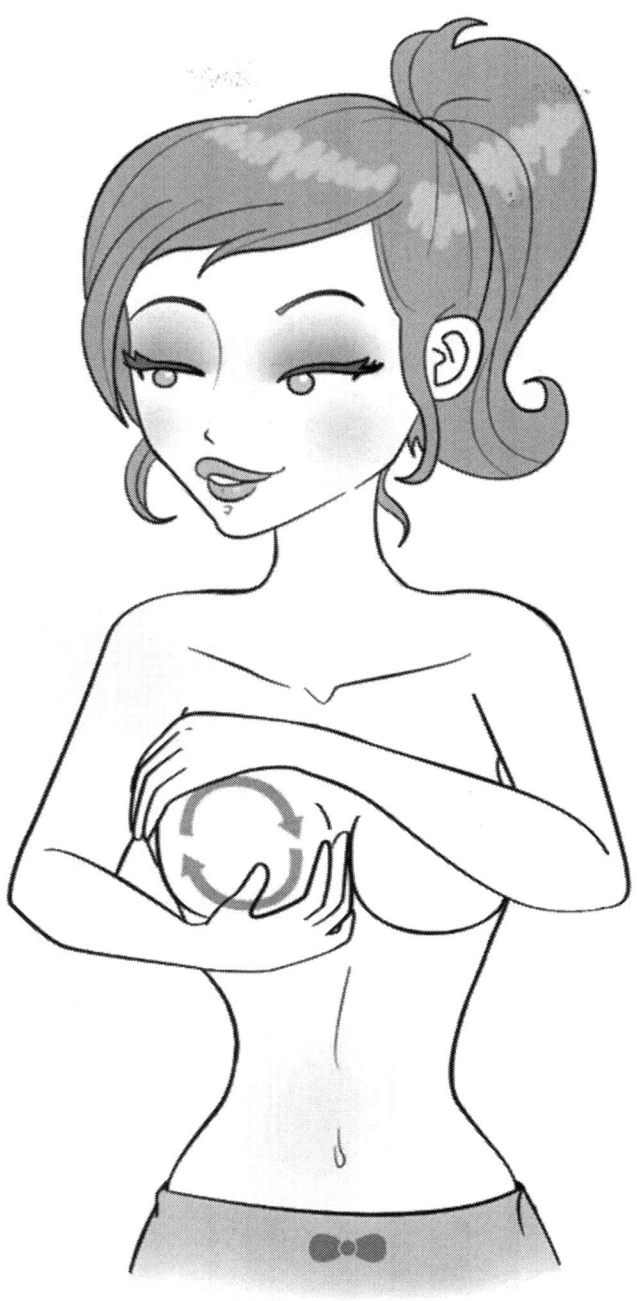

BREAST BOUNCE

Hand position:

One breast at a time - left hand on right breast, right hand on left breast.

Instruction:

1. Lightly cup right hand underneath left breast
2. Gently bounce or jiggle the breast up. This should not be a big motion, just a small, steady motion.
3. Repeat on opposite breast.

Duration:

One minute on each breast.

Notes:

For smaller breasts, bending slightly forward at the waist can make this motion a little easier to perform. For larger breasts, cup the breast with both hands.

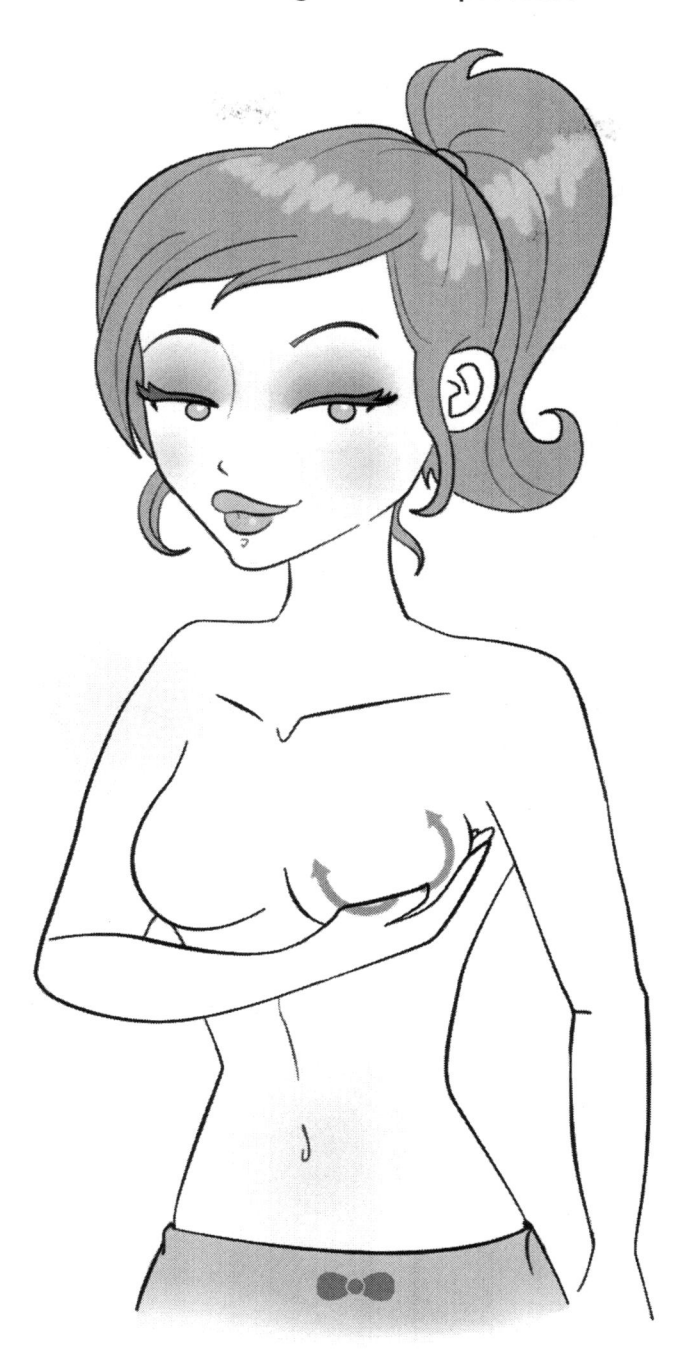

Breast Massage and Acupressure

CHAPTER 3

Acupressure

Acupressure is another self-care technique used to promote breast health and appearance. It is based on the Traditional Chinese Medicine (TCM) practice of acupuncture which dates back thousands of years. While acupuncture uses needles to stimulate a meridian point, also known as an acupoint, these same points can be stimulated with your fingers, knuckles, or palms.

Acupressure is easy to learn, takes only a few minutes a day and can be done virtually anywhere. No special tools are necessary to complete a round of acupressure on yourself and there is no down time as a result of performing acupressure.

HOW DOES ACUPRESSURE WORK?

TCM teaches that life-force energy or Qi (Chi) flows throughout the body and when you are healthy, the energy flows evenly. When this energy flow is blocked or off balance, health issues arise.

The body has 12 major lines (or meridians) of energy running throughout the body. Within these 12 lines are approximately 360 energy points in which needles or finger pressure can be applied to help relieve the blocked energy and bring it back into balance.

Breast Massage and Acupressure

ACUPRESSURE AND BREASTS

Stimulating the meridians associated with the breasts can reap the following benefits:

- Stimulation of the endocrine gland and pituitary glands to release hormones
- Stimulation of breast cells to promote breast development
- Reduced breast pain, mastitis
- Increased lactation
- Alleviation of qi and blood blockages
- Increased circulation and blood flow which results in increased oxygen and nutrients to the chest area
- Elimination of toxins in the chest

HOW TO STIMULATE THE MERIDIAN POINTS

There are three ways you can stimulate a meridian point.

- Apply constant pressure for 1-3 minutes.
- Apply pressure for 5 seconds, release for 5 second. Repeat 10 – 20 times.
- Apply pressure while gently massaging point with small rotations.

You can use your fingers, thumbs, knuckles, or palms to press the meridian point. Some people even use the eraser on a wooden pencil to stimulate the point. For each point, you will want to gently apply enough pressure so there is some discomfort or tenderness at the location of contact, but not too much. Pressing too hard may cause swelling and bruising in the area.

MERIDIAN POINT LOCATIONS ON THE CHEST

Many of the meridian points located on the chest are found between the ribs, also known as intercostal spaces. For example, the 1st intercostal space is the space between the first and second rib. To find the first rib, locate your collarbone and move down until your feel the next

Breast Massage and Acupressure

bone which is your first rib. The 2nd intercostal space is between the second and third rib, etc.

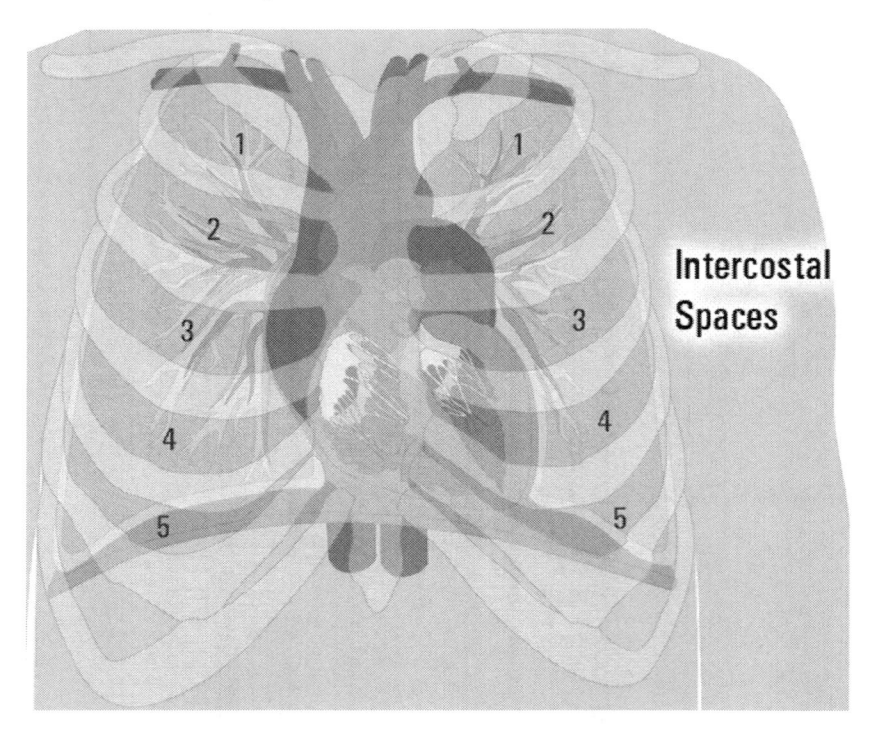

Intercostal Spaces

FINGER MEASUREMENTS

Acupressure point locations are generally measured by cun, a traditional Chinese unit of length. Common cun measurements used for acupressure point locations include:

- 1 cun - the width of a person's thumb at the knuckle.
- 1.5 cun - the width of the middle and index fingers at the knuckle.
- 2 cun - the width of the person's index, middle, and ring fingers at the knuckle
- 3 cun - the width of the person's four fingers at the knuckle.

Breast Massage and Acupressure

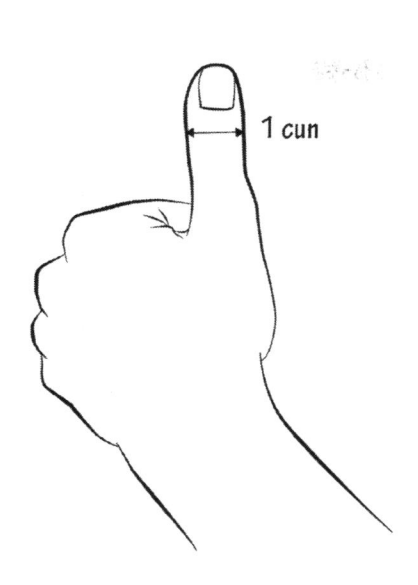

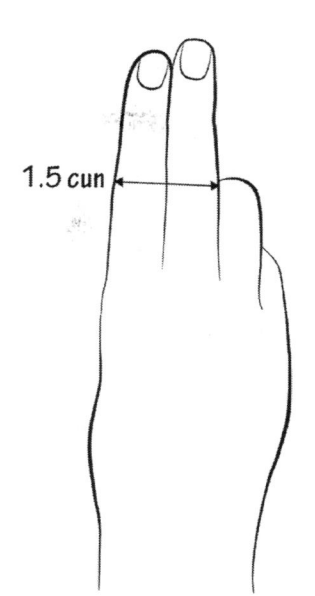

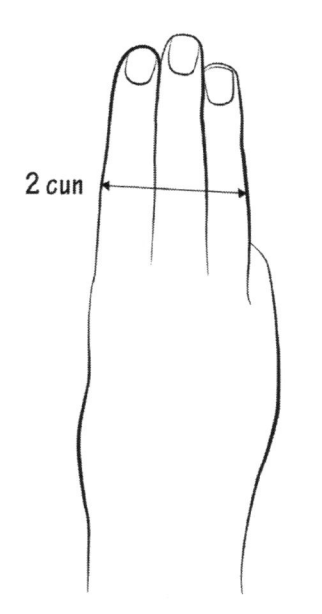

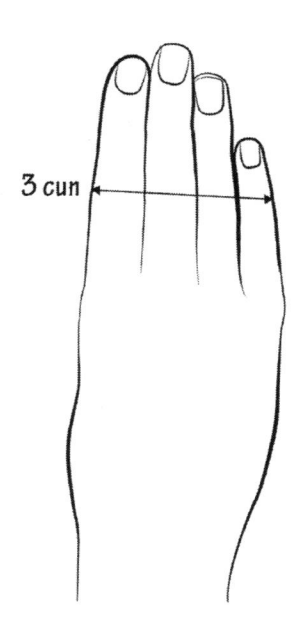

1 cun

1.5 cun

2 cun

3 cun

Breast Massage and Acupressure

ACUPRESSURE TIPS

- Don't worry too much about hitting the acupressure point exactly. Pressing the general area can be effective as well.
- Most of the points found in this book are bilateral, meaning they can be found on both the right side and left side of the body. For these points, you can press the right and left sides at the same time if positioning allows or you can press them individually.
- Acupressure can be done anytime and anywhere, so take advantage of its simplicity. Press the points while watching TV, using the computer, or talking on the phone. If you are out in public, you can easily spend a little time on points like the Shao Ze point (page 39) located on the pinky finger or the Nei Guan point (page 40) located near the wrist, without getting any weird looks.
- There are seven main acupoints that are beneficial for the breasts but there are also additional points later in the book that are beneficial. It is recommended that you do the seven main points, if possible, which only take a few minutes to complete. The acupoints listed in this book do not have to be done in the order presented.

CHAPTER 4

Acupressure Points

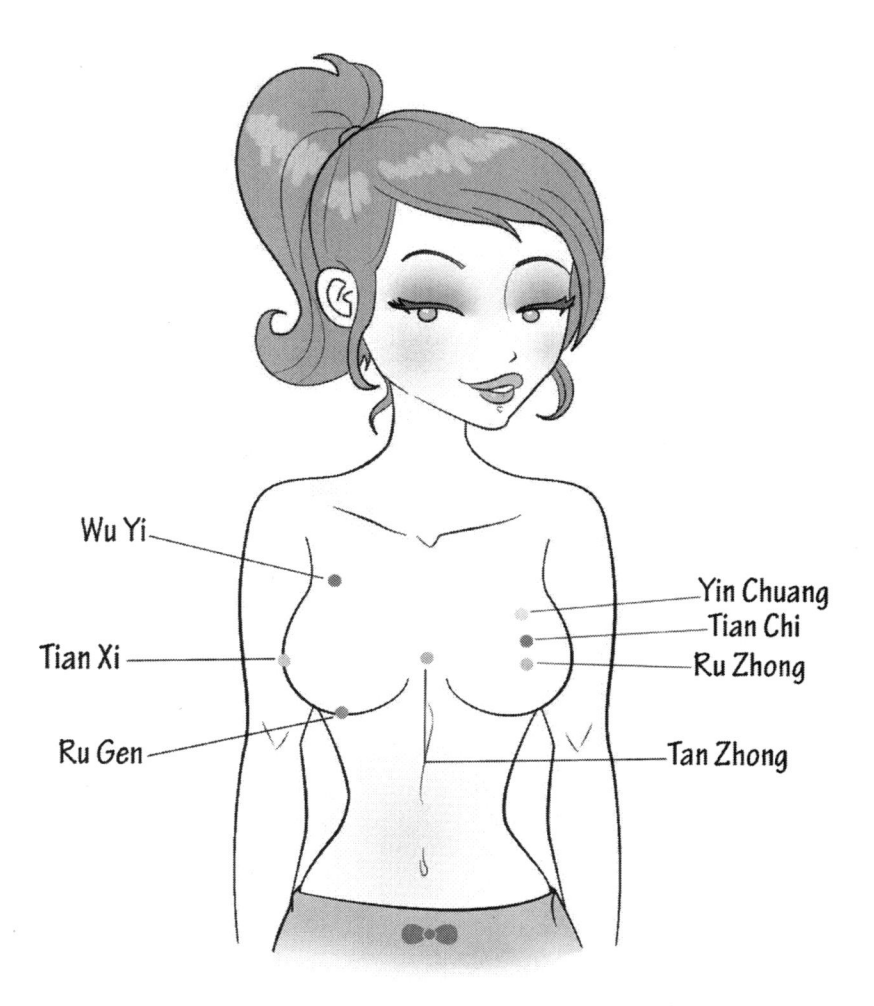

Wu Yi

Tian Xi

Ru Gen

Yin Chuang
Tian Chi
Ru Zhong

Tan Zhong

The following acupressure techniques are not recommended for women who are pregnant. Many of the points described may induce labor.

TAN ZHONG POINT - 膻中

Translation:

Chest Center

Meridian:

Conception Vessel (CV 17 / Ren 17)

Location:

Middle of chest between nipples.

Function:
- treatment of mastitis, abscess, and breast pain
- promotes lactation
- regulates lung qi
- increases and purifies blood supply
- energizes and increases circulation in chest

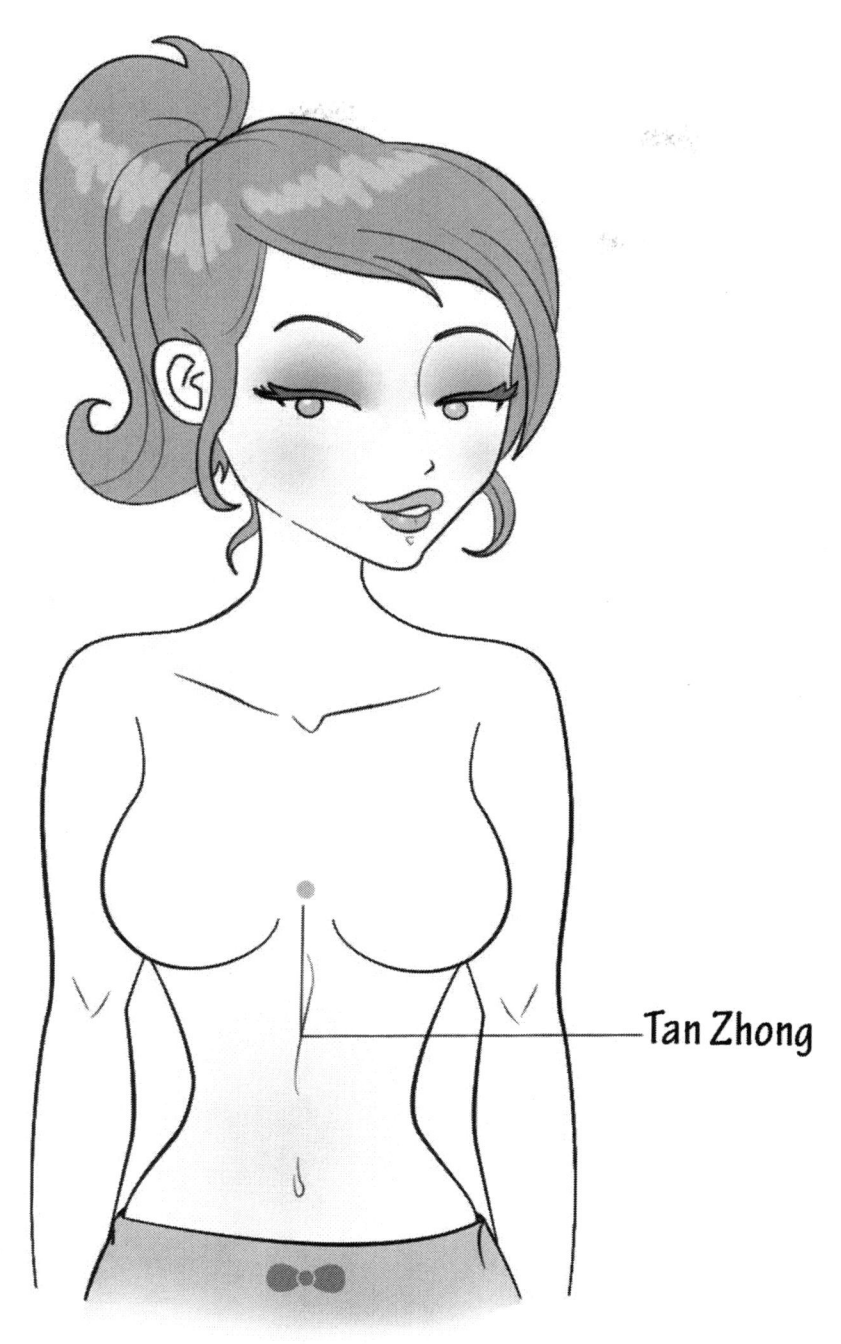

Breast Massage and Acupressure

Tan Zhong

TIAN CHI POINT - 膻中

Translation:

Heavenly Pool

Meridian:

Pericardium (PC1)

Location:

1 cun outside of nipple on 4th intercostal space.

Function:
- increases lactation
- regulates qi
- treats disorders of the breast due to stagnant qi and blood, including breast pain, swelling, mastitis, and abscess

Breast Massage and Acupressure

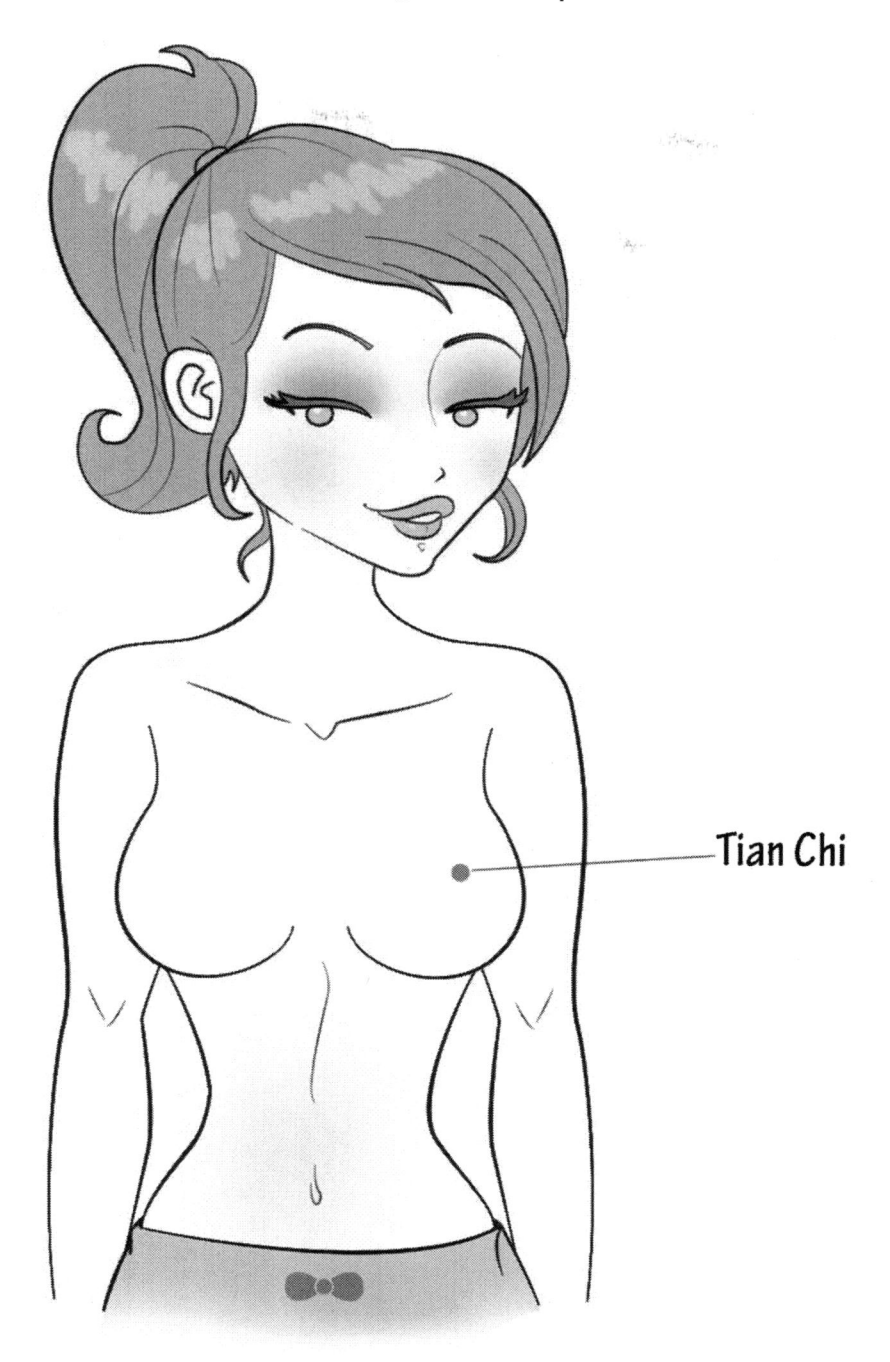

Tian Chi

43

TIAN XI POINT - 天谿

Translation:

Heavenly Creek

Meridian:

Spleen (SP18)

Location:

6 cun from chest center.

Function:
- breast development
- treatment of breast pain and acute mastitis
- increases lactation
- relieves breast congestion
- relieves qi stagnation in the chest

Breast Massage and Acupressure

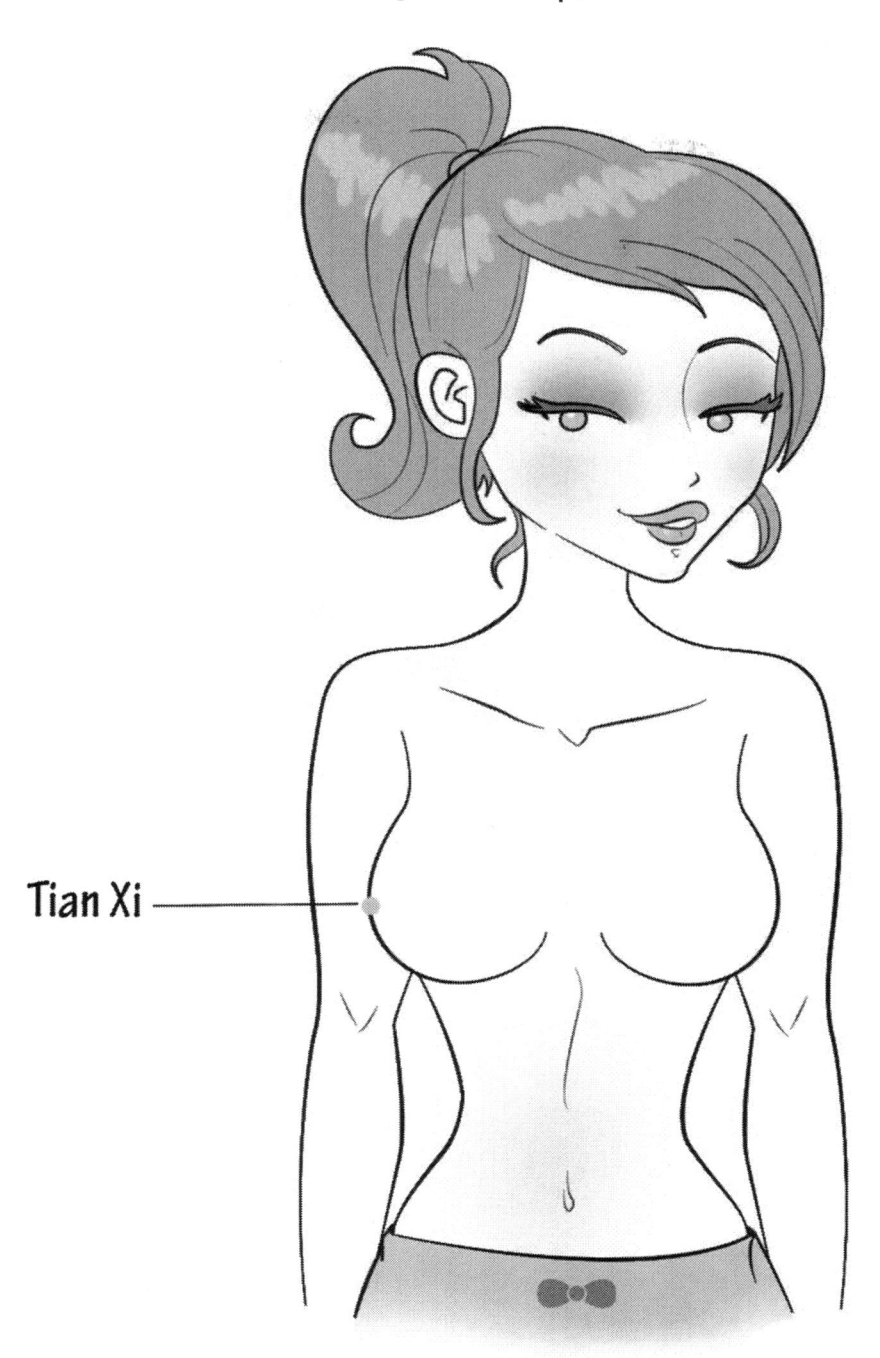

Tian Xi

45

WU YI POINT - 屋翳

Translation:

Roof

Meridian:

Stomach (ST15)

Location:

Above the nipples on 2nd intercostal space.

Function:
- breast augmentation
- treatment for insufficient secretion of milk, and breast pain
- helps to normalize the qi and blood circulation of the breast

Breast Massage and Acupressure

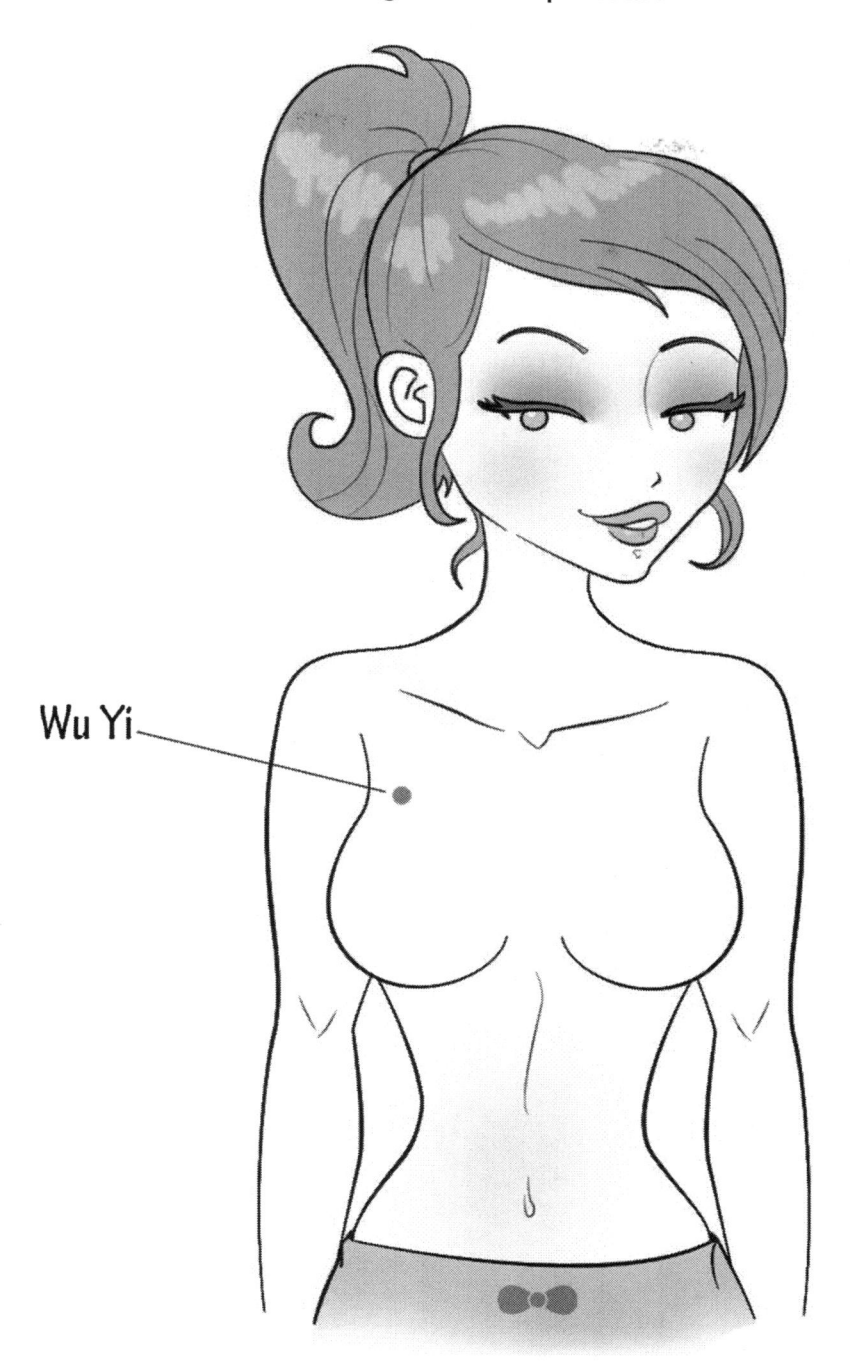

Wu Yi

47

YING CHUANG POINT - 膺窗

Translation:

Breast Window

Meridian:

Stomach (ST 16)

Location:

Above the nipple on 3rd intercostal space.

Function:
- benefits overall breast health
- treatment for mastitis and breast abscess
- relieves breast tenderness, pain, and swelling
- improves lactation

Breast Massage and Acupressure

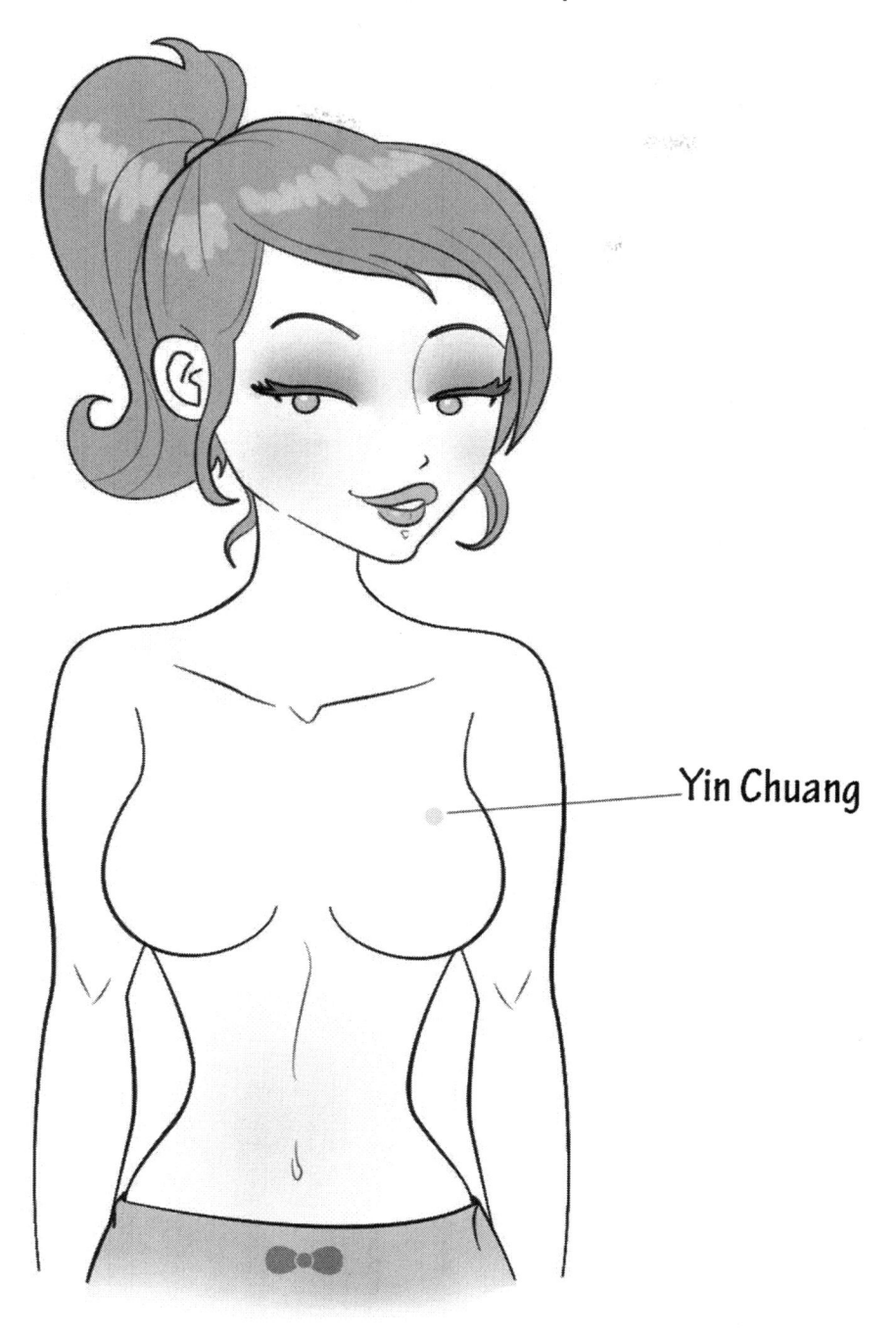

Yin Chuang

49

RU ZHONG POINT - 乳中

Translation:

Breast Center

Meridian:

Stomach (ST17)

Location:

Center of the nipple.

Function:
- Improves hormone levels; treats hormone imbalances

Note:

Generally used as a reference point in acupuncture and not stimulated with needles. Pressure does not need to be applied. It can be stimulated by touch.

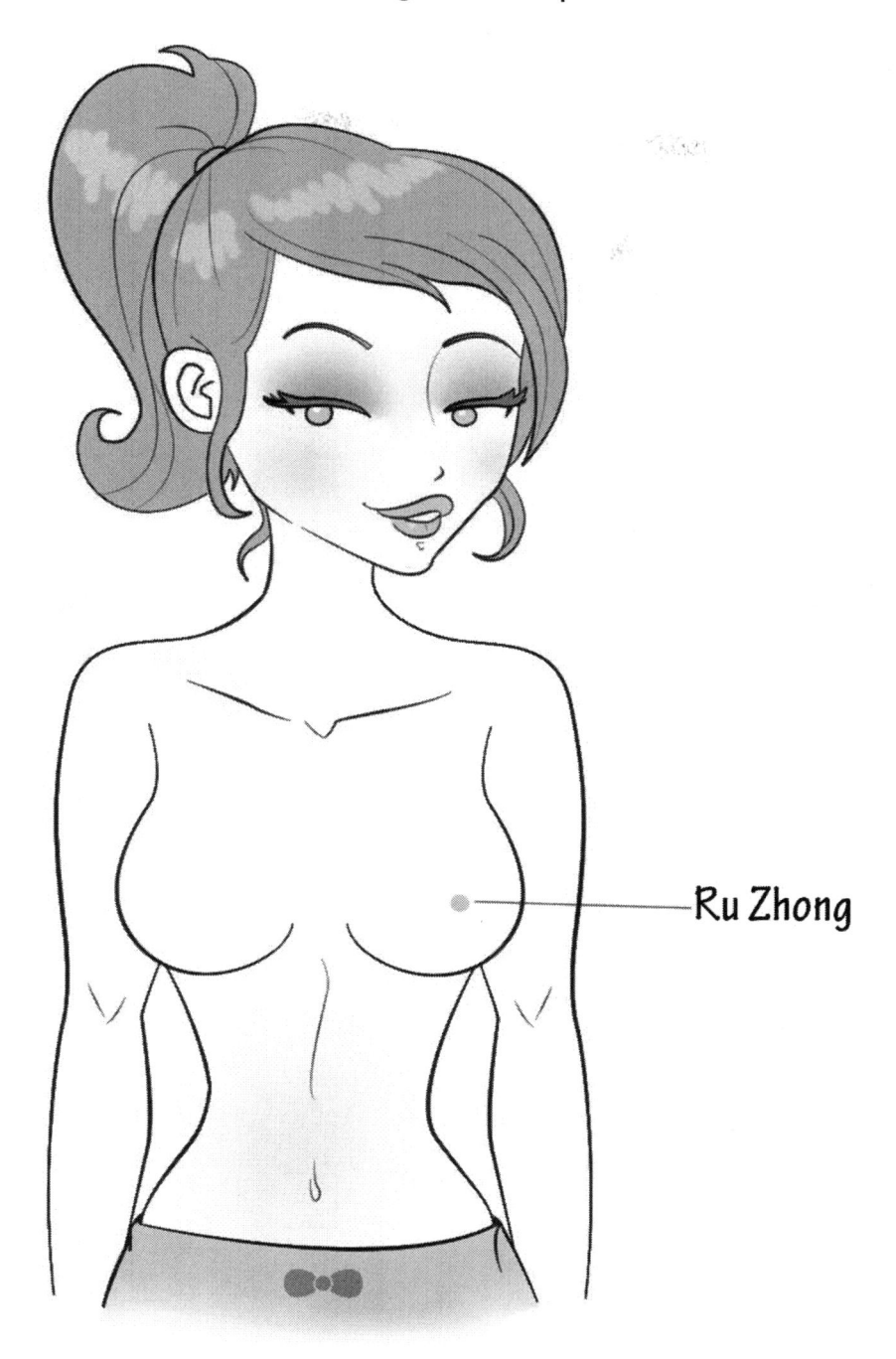

Breast Massage and Acupressure

Ru Zhong

RU GEN POINT - 乳根

Translation:

Breast Root

Meridian:

Stomach (ST18)

Location:

Directly below nipple on 5th intercostal space.

Function:
- increases the secretion of milk
- helps with breast development and growth
- treatment of many disorders of the mammary glands, including mastitis
- relieves breast tension, pain, and swelling

Note:

Major point for many breast disorders / important local point for treating breast diseases and insufficient lactation.

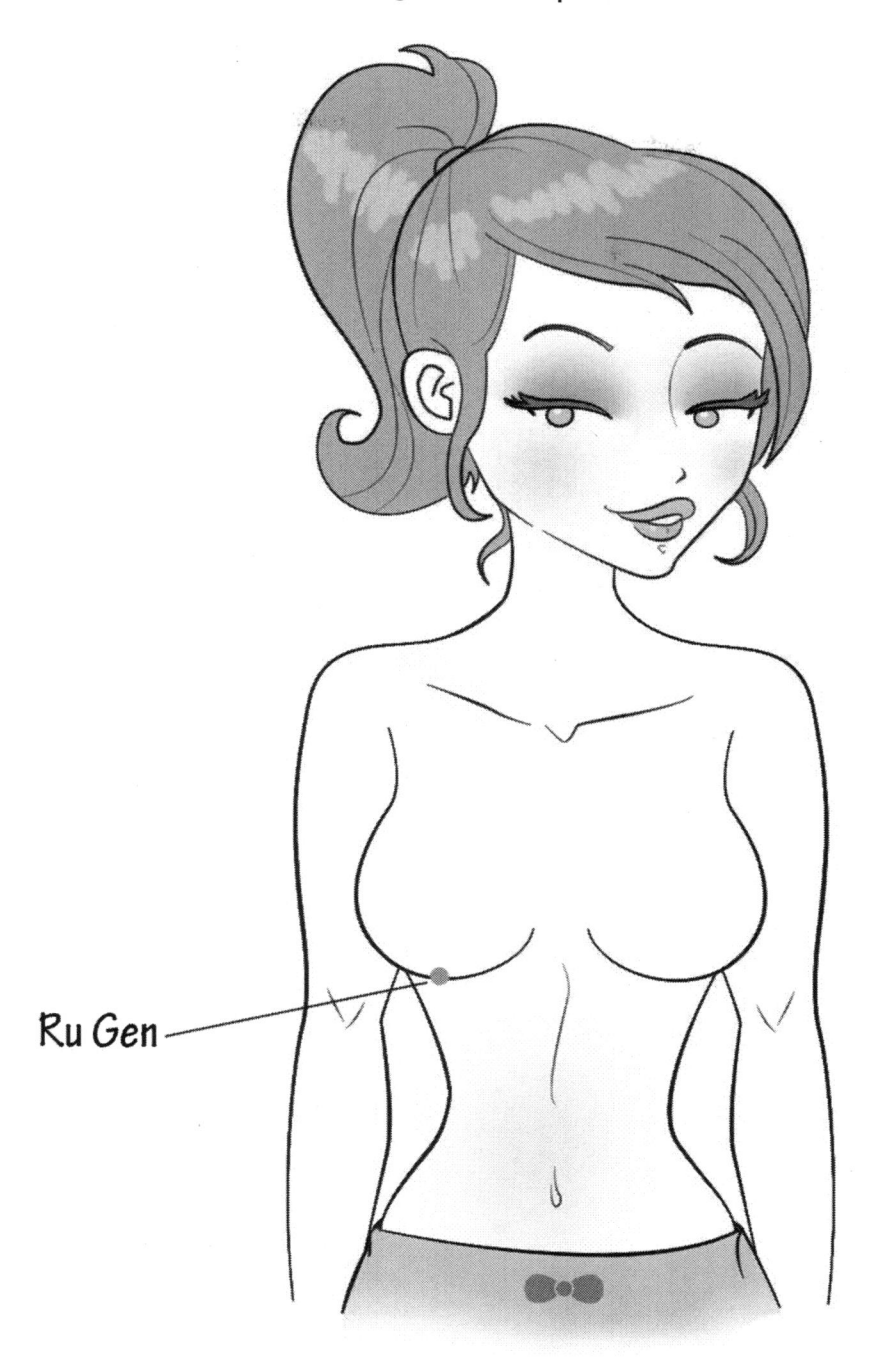

Breast Massage and Acupressure

Ru Gen

53

CHAPTER 5

More Acupressure Points

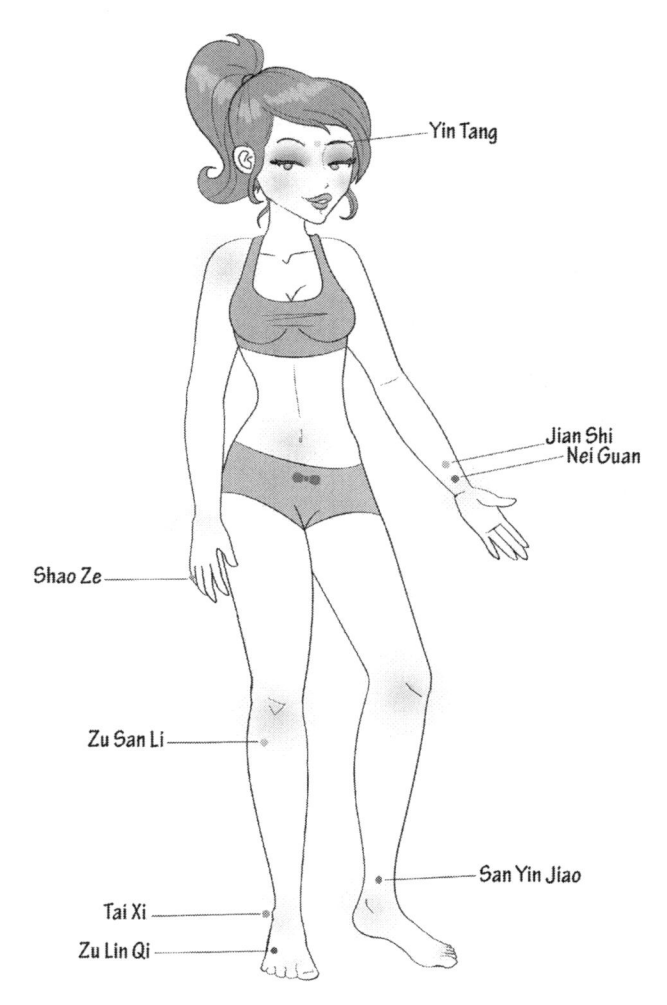

The following acupressure techniques are not recommended for women who are pregnant. Many of the points described may induce labor.

YIN TANG POINT - 印堂

Translation:

Hall of Seal

Meridian:

Miscellaneous Point (MHN3) / Forehead Point

Location:

Between inner side of eyebrows.

Function:

Stimulates pituitary gland and improves endocrine functions; regulates and balances hormones

Breast Massage and Acupressure

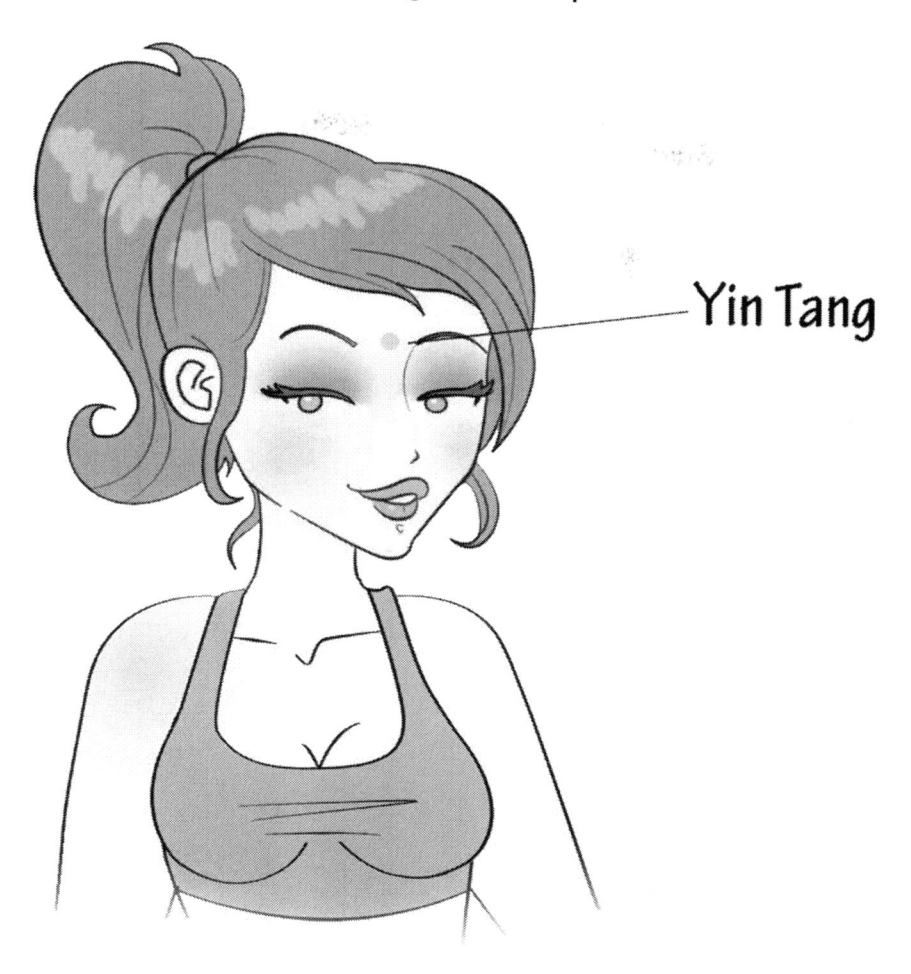

Yin Tang

SHAO ZE POINT - 少澤

Translation:

Lesser Marsh

Meridian:

Small Intestine (SI1)

Location:

Bottom corner of the fingernail on the outside edge of little finger/pinky finger.

Function:
- stimulates breast blood circulation
- stimulates breast tissue, helps develop the chest
- increases the production and flow of breast milk

Breast Massage and Acupressure

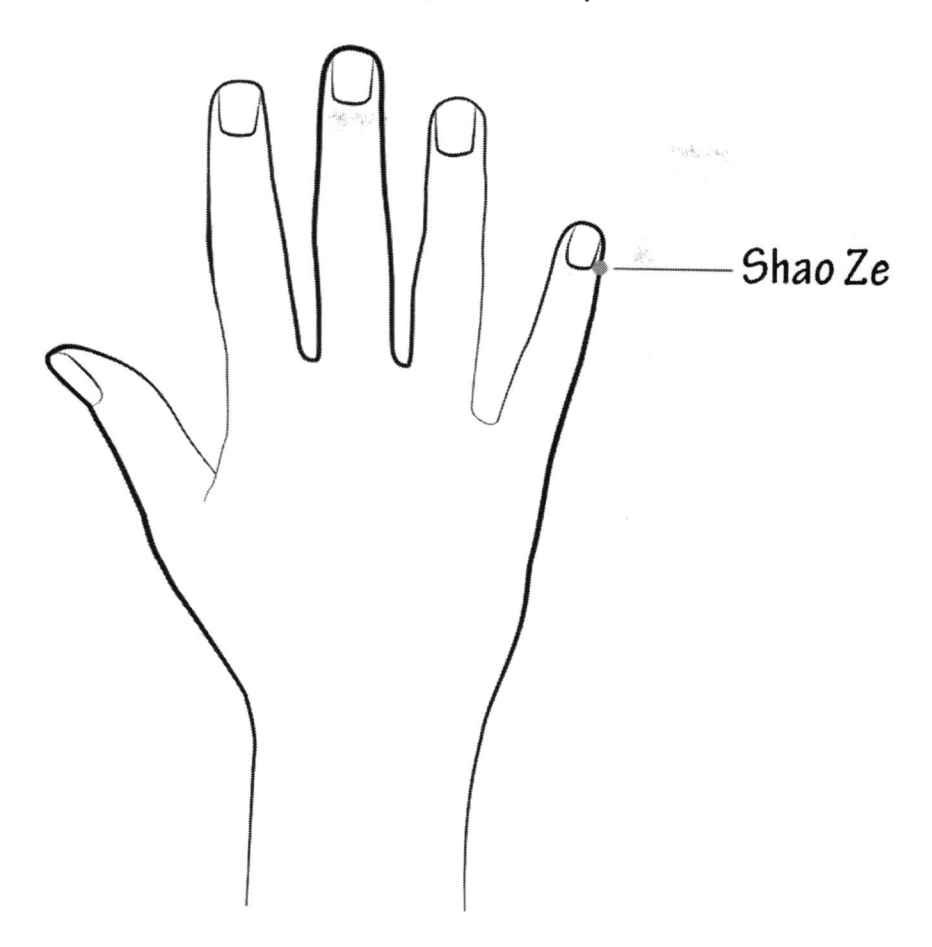

Shao Ze

NEI GUAN POINT - 內關

Translation:

Leg Three Miles

Meridian:

Stomach (ST36)

Location:

3 cun below the knee cap on the outer side of the leg bone between shinbone and muscle.

Function:
- regulates qi and blood
- increases nutrient absorption
- strengthens reproductive system
- treats for acute mastitis
- improves circulation in the whole body

Breast Massage and Acupressure

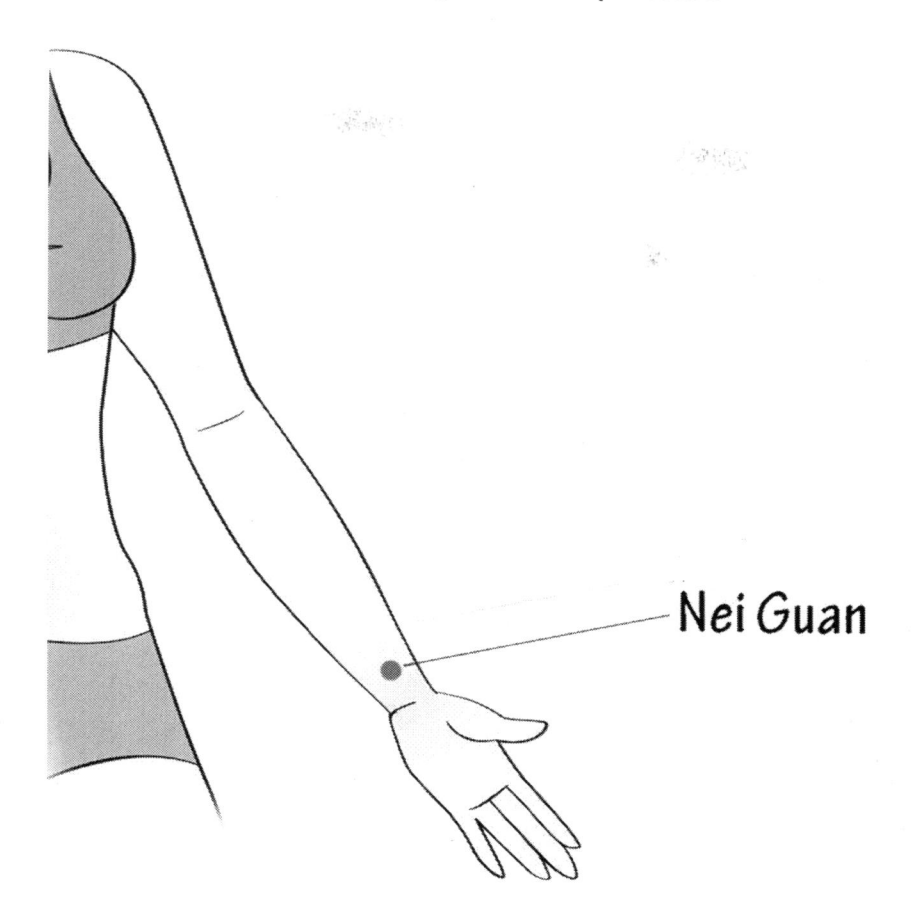

Nei Guan

SAN YIN JIAO POINT - 三陰交

Translation:

Three Yin Intersection

Meridian:

Spleen (SP6)

Location:

On the inside of leg, 3 cun up from the center of ankle bone.

Function:
- regulates hormones
- regulates menstruation; relieves PMS symptoms
- tones and strengthens uterus
- induces labor
- promotes fertility
- helps body absorb nutrients

Breast Massage and Acupressure

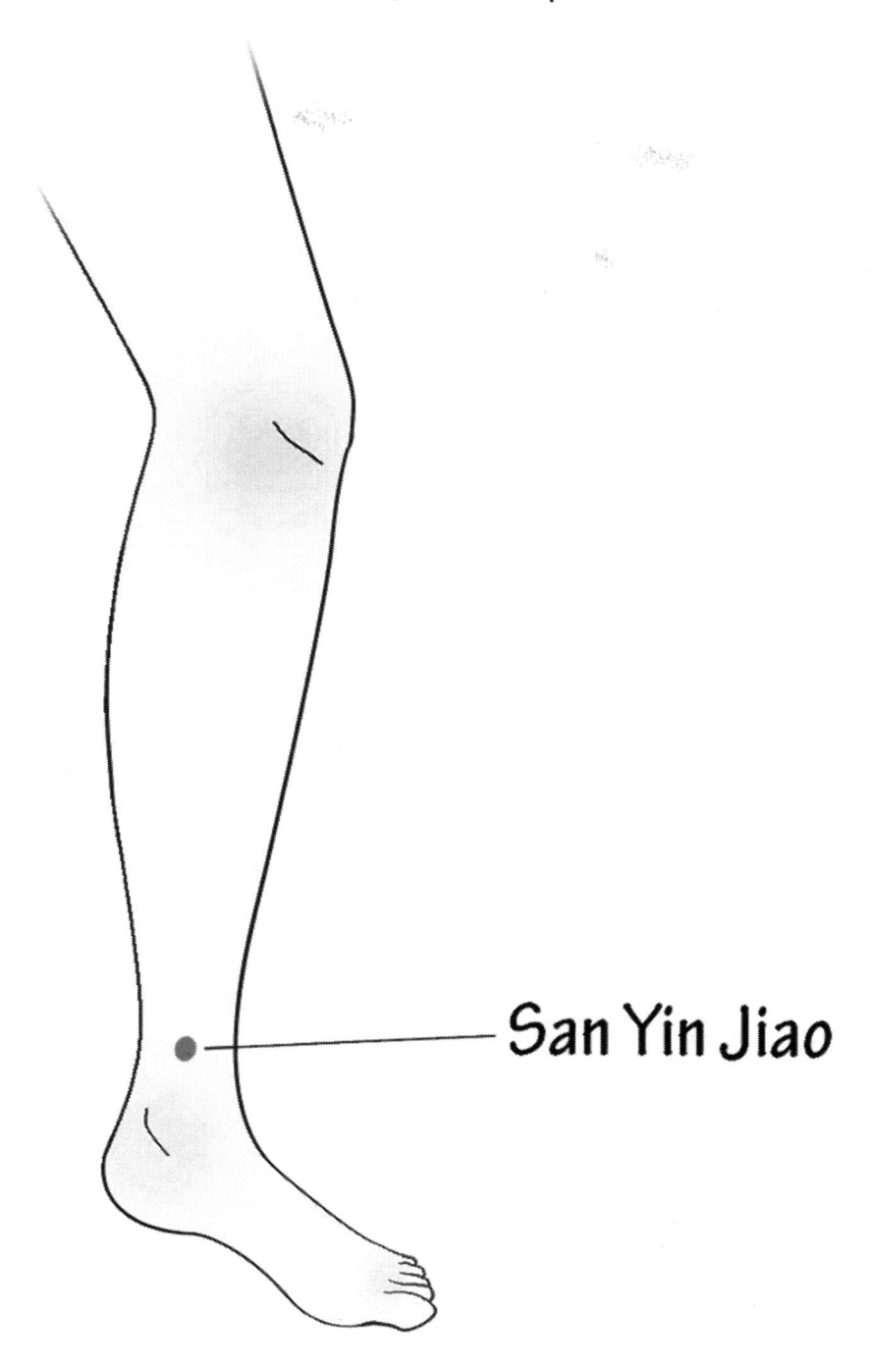

San Yin Jiao

TAI XI POINT - 大鐘

Translation:

Great Stream

Meridian:

Kidney (KD3)

Location:

On the inside of the ankle, located in the depression between the ankle bone and Achilles tendon.

Functions:
- promotes good hormonal balance
- strengthens kidneys, adrenals and reproductive system
- aids in fertility
- relives labor pains

Added bonus: promotes healthy hair growth.

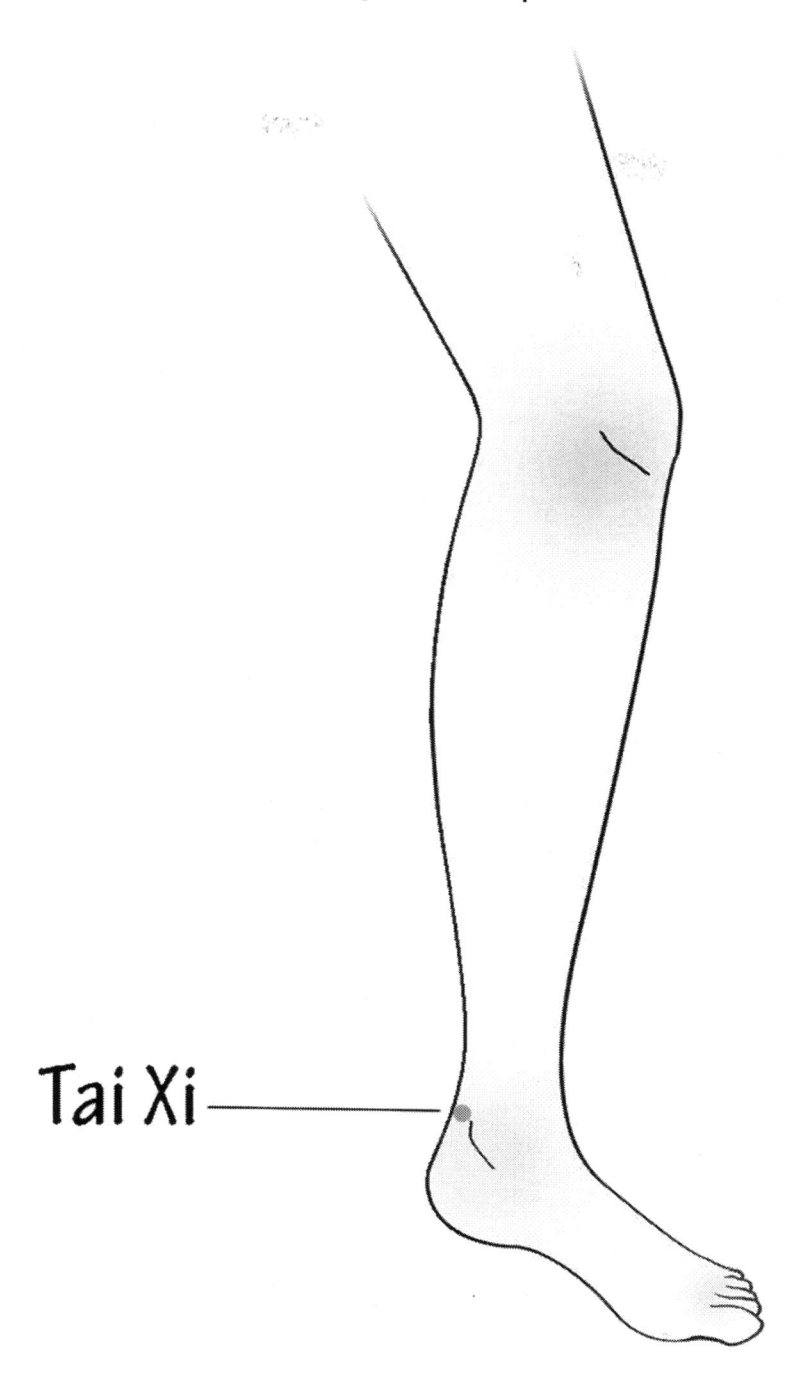

Breast Massage and Acupressure

Tai Xi

JIAN SHI POINT - 間使

Translation:

Intermediary Messenger

Meridian:

Pericardium (P5)

Location:

Inner arm, 3 cun up from the wrist crease in between tendons.

Function:
- regulates chest qi
- regulates menstruation

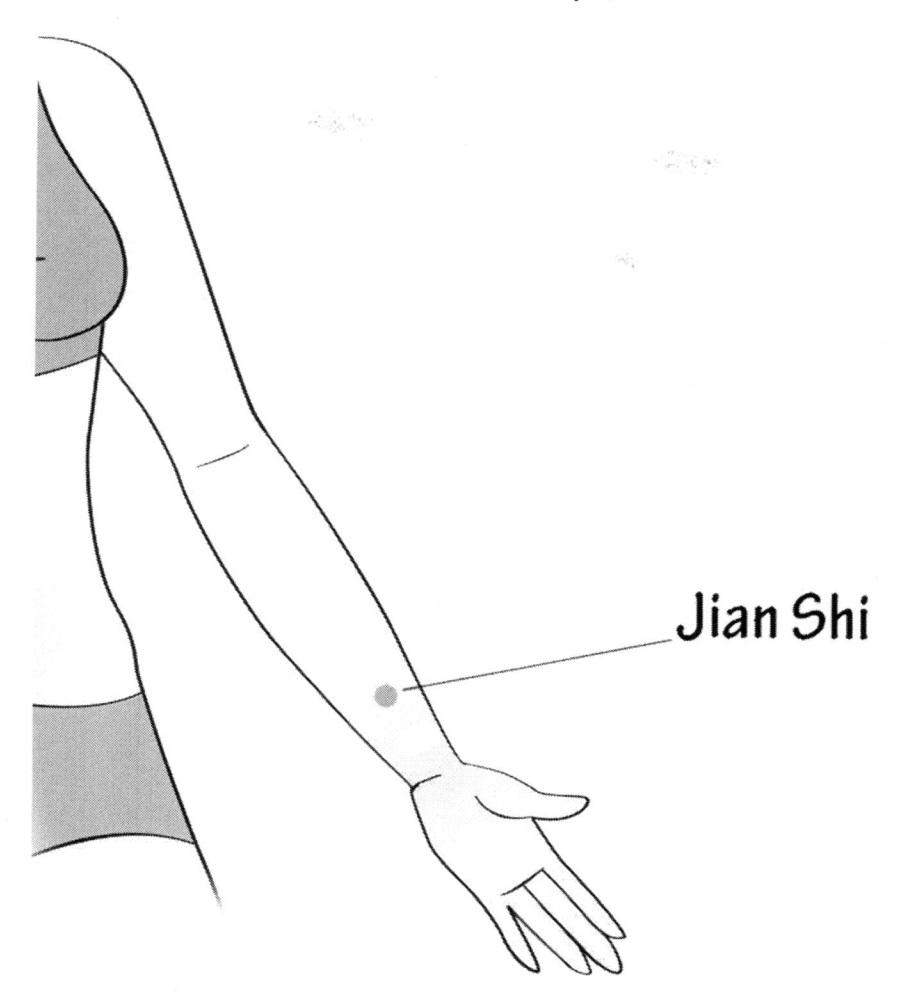

Breast Massage and Acupressure

Jian Shi

ZU LIN QI POINT - 足臨泣

Translation:

Foot Falling Tears

Meridian:

Gall Bladder (GB 41)

Location:

Top of foot just above where the fourth and fifth (pinky) toe come together and form a "V".

Function:
- treatment of mastitis and breast distention, pain, and abscesses
- irregular menstruation

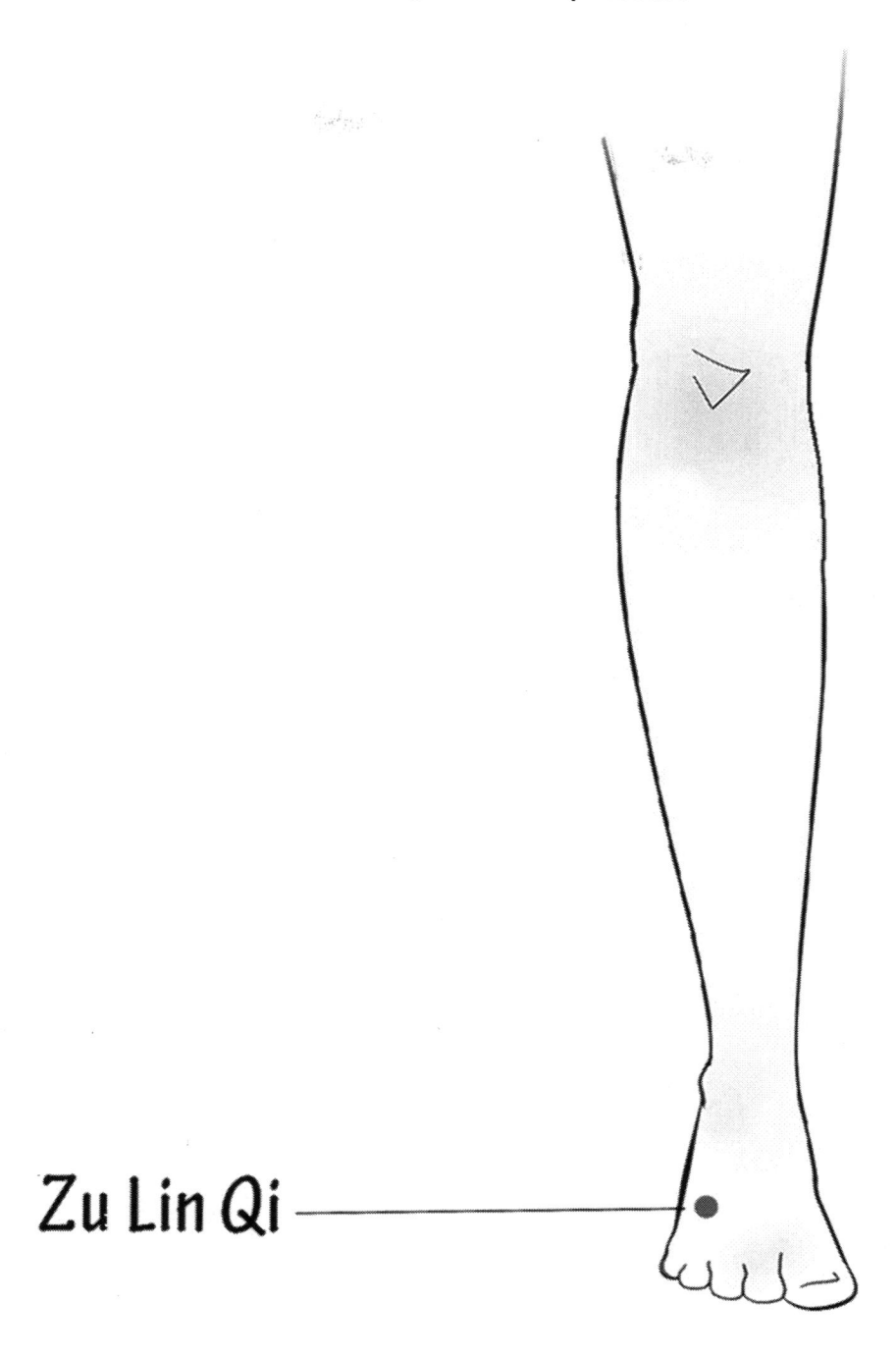

Breast Massage and Acupressure

Zu Lin Qi

Sample Massage + Acupressure Regimen

MASSAGE TECHNIQUES

Cleavage Push	10 times
Breast Circles	10 times outward
Breast Swirls	20 times inward
Cleavage Glide	20 times
Nipple Grab	20 times
Knead Some Boobs	50 times

ACUPRESSURE POINTS (PRESS AND RELEASE TECHNIQUE)

Tian Xi	10 - 20 times
Ru Gen	10 - 20 times
Tian Chi	10 - 20 times
Tan Zhong	10 - 20 times

Breast Massage and Acupressure

BOOKS BY ALEXA REYNA

Breast Enhancement Secrets and Myths from Around the World

Beginner's Guide to Natural Breast Enlargement

A Crash Course in Growing Breasts Naturally

Made in the USA
Middletown, DE
22 May 2018